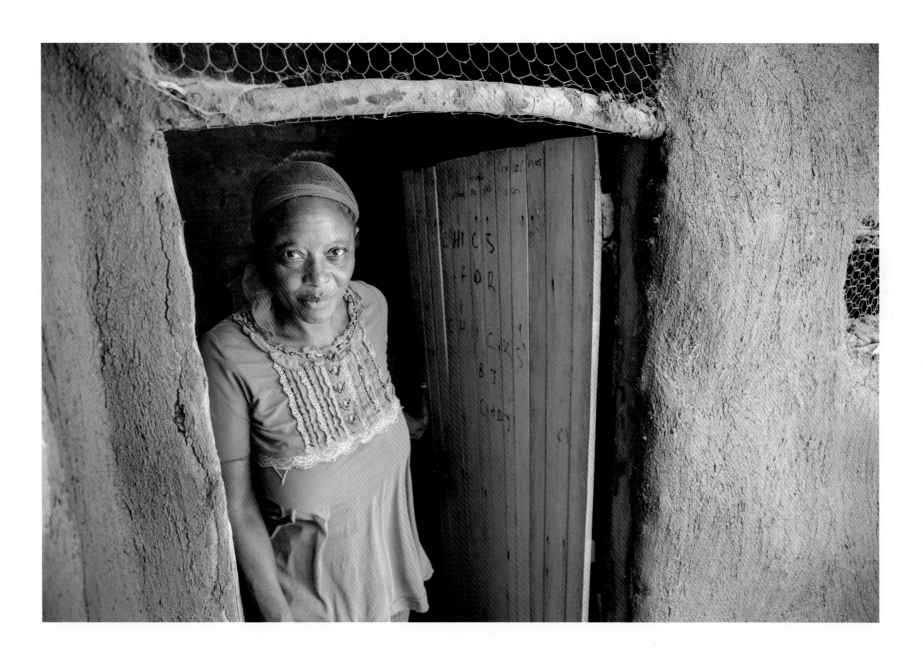

From AIDS to POPULATION HEALTH

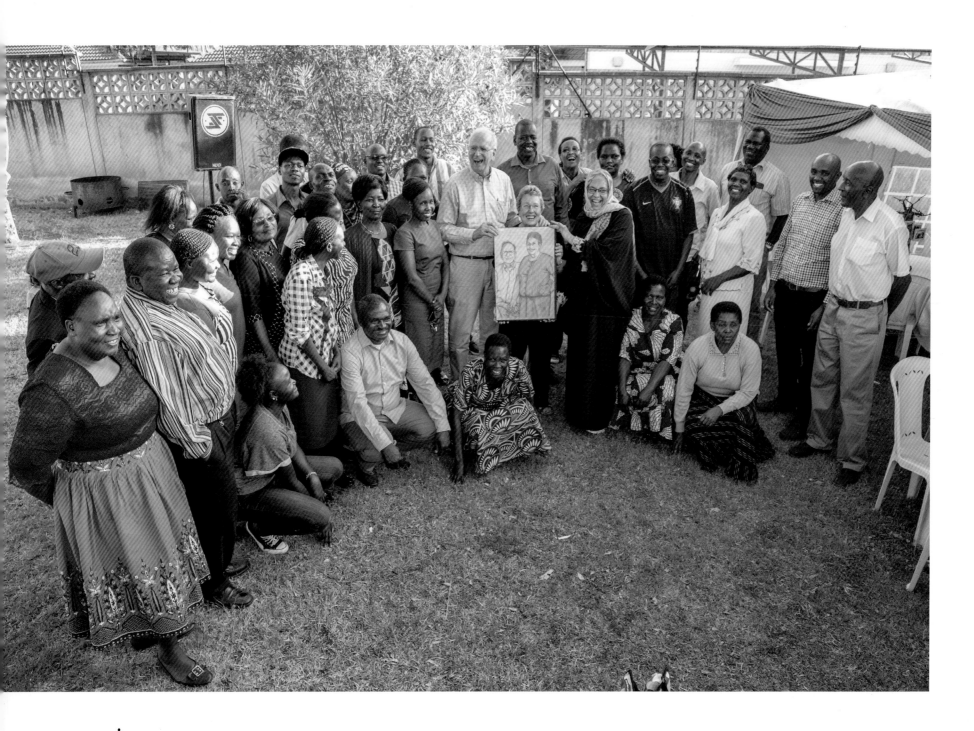

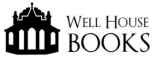

WELL HOUSE
BOOKS

The IU House family celebrated 20 years with Joe and Sarah Ellen Mamlin in the garden of Hilltop House with food and dance on March 16, 2019. The staff gave the Mamlins a portrait that now hangs on the wall of the dining room.

From AIDS to POPULATION HEALTH

How an American University and a Kenyan Medical School Transformed Healthcare in East Africa

Text and photos by JAMES D. KELLY

INDIANA UNIVERSITY PRESS

This book is a publication of

Indiana University Press
Office of Scholarly Publishing
Herman B Wells Library 350
1320 East 10th Street
Bloomington, Indiana 47405 USA

iupress.org

Manufactured in Korea

First printing 2022

Library of Congress Cataloging-in-Publication Data

Names: Kelly, James D., [date] author.
Title: From AIDS to population health : how
    an American university and a Kenyan
    medical school transformed healthcare
    in East Africa / James D. Kelly.
Identifiers: LCCN 2022024169 (print) | LCCN
    2022024170 (ebook) | ISBN 9780253062758
    (cloth) | ISBN 9780253062765 (pdf)
Subjects: LCSH: AMPATH. | Health services
    administration—Kenya. | Medical care—Kenya.
Classification: LCC RA971 .K439135 2022 (print) | LCC
    RA971 (ebook) | DDC 362.1068—dc23/eng/20220523
LC record available at https://lccn.loc.gov/2022024169
LC ebook record available at https://
lccn.loc.gov/2022024170

*Dedicated to the staff members who each day give life and meaning
to the Academic Model Providing Access to Healthcare (AMPATH)
by leading with care for the people of Kenya.*

CONTENTS

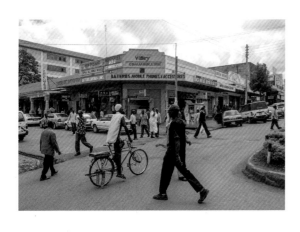 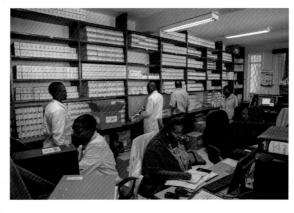

PART ONE
INTRODUCTION

PART TWO
PHOTOGRAPHIC ESSAYS OF WORKERS

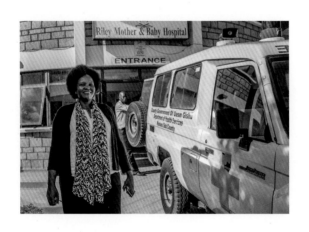

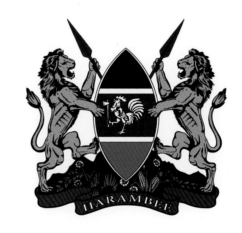

PART THREE
LEADERSHIP PROFILES

PART FOUR
RESEARCH

PREFACE

I AM TRYING TO PAY A debt. I have been privileged to visit with the people of Eldoret, Kenya, for nearly a dozen years now. I say "privileged" because it has been an honor and pleasure to know the people of AMPATH but also because I have taken advantage of an entitlement that white people enjoy. I do not know why I was born white in the United States instead of Black in Africa, but I do recognize that the circumstances of my birth have afforded me opportunity I have not earned and that I need to pay for it if the world is to be made right.

My privilege derives from a long history of people who trace their ancestry to Europe subjugating the people who trace their ancestry to Africa. As an American, I enjoy a life purchased with the labor stolen from enslaved people whose ancestors were stolen from Africa. As a professor at Indiana University, I teach my students on land stolen from Indigenous people recognized now as Miami, Delaware, Potawatomi, and Shawnee. We call our

state Indiana, a tacit if largely unrealized acknowledgment that our home was someone else's home before us. This theft by my ancestors provided great economic gains that I continue to benefit from.

Shortly after graduating from Indiana University with my doctoral degree, I had the great personal fortune to wander into a meeting room in a hotel I was staying at in Chicago. The Reverend Jesse Jackson was addressing a crowd with an oratory style that now reminds me of the great speakers I have since listened to in Kenya, Uganda, Tanzania, and Ethiopia. At the time, though, I thought of him as simply a Black American. Sure, he had just run for president, but I was not thinking of him as a son of Africa. I had not yet deeply considered the relationship he and all Black Americans have to a continent on the other side of the ocean that few will ever see but that is a part of them nevertheless. At the time, I had never visited Africa and didn't know any Africans. But what Reverend Jackson said that afternoon in 1991 changed my way of thinking and has continued to resonate as I have photographed and written this book.

He explained that white people living today did not own slaves, did not colonize Africa, and did not displace the Native Americans. He nevertheless said that reparations ought to be paid, not just to American Blacks but also to the African nations from which they were stolen. "The voices that cry out for reparations have been seen as marginal or radical, but they cry for justice," he said. "What is America willing to do to repair the damage done?" He said the government ought to make the payments and acknowledged that such a day might never come, "but at the very least, white people can acknowledge that they owe a debt." Since that day I have tried to do a wee bit more than what Jackson said was "the very least."

I do acknowledge the debt my European ancestors owe to the people of Africa and America. I myself cannot pay it back. It is too large. No amount of money is sufficient to compensate for the millions of lives lived in shackles and without their loved ones and their land. I cannot undo what has been done. None of us can. But I can use my privilege to help tell the story that Reverend Jackson taught me about in Chicago.

I am still faced with an impossible task. The story you need to hear, need to know, and need to understand—well, it is not my story. It is a Kenyan story. It is a story about Kenyans building a healthcare system in the wake of generations of colonial exploitation. It is a story about those Kenyans fighting the HIV virus, and it is a story about those Kenyans expanding upon the lessons they learned from that great nation-building effort so that all Kenyans can live healthy, sustainable lives. It is a story surely better told by a Kenyan voice than by mine, but here I am, using my privilege to tell someone else's story.

This is what journalists do. They find a story that isn't being told loudly enough and try to tell it themselves. It is an imperfect attempt every time. We listen, we watch, and we do what we can to understand, but in the end, we are telling stories that others have lived and that they understand in ways we never will. I get to try because I have been given opportunity to try. Instead of paying those reparations, my government paid me to go to Africa to teach Kenyan students about journalism and to create a truthful story that describes a thirty-year partnership between people in Kenya and people in Indiana. It is the very least my government could do, and it is the very least I could do.

This book is an imperfect, inadequate attempt to pay a monstrous debt. I believe real monetary reparations are owed, and I hope the story I tell in these pages lets Kenyans know we are trying and lets Americans know we need to do more.

What is good and right and just is that ever since that day I stood in the back of the room listening to Jesse Jackson, Hoosiers have been working with Kenyans as if they were brothers and sisters. Hoosiers have used their privilege to live in the Great Rift Valley, and they have used their privilege to bring Kenyans to the homes they have made on Native American land. Every time I have looked at AMPATH since first going to Eldoret in 2009, I have seen friendship, respect, admiration, and love.

I cannot let this story go. It must be told. If I have done anything right, it is because my Kenyan friends have helped me see, helped me understand, and helped me tell their story back to them. If it rings at all true to their ears, it is because I have been a good student. Their ability and willingness to teach me has only added to the debt I owe Black people who trace their ancestors to Africa.

ACKNOWLEDGMENTS

I OWE THIS BOOK TO THESE fine folks. I had help writing this book. A lot of help from a lot of people living in a lot of different places. This is where I acknowledge their kind assistance. I'm going to miss someone and likely get the order of importance wrong too, so bear with me.

Carol Ann Kelly helped the most. For all of our thirty-three years together, she has cared for my children and me as I took off for overseas places about one month of every year. She tells wonderful stories, and many of them begin with, "Well, Jim was out of the country when . . ." There were sick babies, broken cars, ice storms, smoke alarms, snow days, and bumps in the night. Her stories were always funny, but they were about what happened when I was away. This book is about what happened when she was away with me in Africa. She retired early from a job she loved so she could live in servants' quarters in a small city on the other side of the planet. Eldoret was very familiar to me, but it was literally a world away from what she knew. Every day while we were in the IU House, she listened to me tell tales about who I had met and what I had seen. She calmed me down every time I decided nothing was going to work, and she celebrated every time something did, in fact, work. It was our big adventure. Since then she has read drafts of proposals, letters, budgets, chapters, and more chapters. She's the best proofreader I know. In other words, she has kept me focused and accurate.

Those children Carol cared for while I was away also helped me with this book. Both Anna and Megan read early drafts and provided insightful feedback that helped me land the Fulbright award and the book contract. They visited us in Eldoret and reminded me all over again just how special the Great Rift Valley is by their constant joy over being there with their parents and meeting my friends, and they told me how nice it was to see me in the place they had long imagined me in before.

Now the order of importance becomes a little less certain. Abraham Kiprop Mulwo; his wife, Monicah Oroiyo; and their children, Cynthia, Diana, and Kigen, welcomed me back to Kenya after a seven-year absence. They welcomed Carol and me into their home the evening after our arrival. At the time they were the parents of two daughters, and we reveled in their good luck because we have always thought two girls made for the perfect family. But they taught us that three was wonderful too when Monicah delivered a son midway through our time in Eldoret. Not only did their family's hospitality sustain us during our stay in Kenya, but Abraham's support allowed me to teach at Moi University and land the Fulbright in the first place. *Ngudu.*

Others also assisted me with the landing. Sylvester Kimaiyo has four times now granted me the permission I needed to tell stories about AMPATH. Thrice he invited my students to interview folks at AMPATH, and the last time he gave me unfettered access to literally everyone in the organization. Similarly, Bob Einterz has four times lent his unqualified support to my efforts to tell AMPATH stories. He encouraged me to bring students, wrote an embarrassingly generous letter supporting my Fulbright application, and always greeted me as if I was doing him a favor when it was I who benefited from his largess. Joe Mamlin has also given me everything I have asked for during the decade I have been asking him for favors. I think his wife, Sarah Ellen, influences him on my account. She helped me find my way during my scouting trip a decade ago, and ever since, the two of them have provided warm conversation and steadfast support to my students and me. Obi Okumu-Bigambo first gave me reason to believe I could share AMPATH's story. Within an hour of arriving at the IU House for the first time in 2009, Obi was there telling me "we can do it"—even before I had laid out my plan. His optimism and faith in me and all his students have buoyed me countless times over our years of friendship. At home in Indiana, Brad Hamm first told me of AMPATH. He supported my plans to teach IU and Moi students in Kenya and helped me secure my Fulbright award. Were it not for him, I might still not know about the amazing partnership in Eldoret.

These leaders have been important to me as I have worked to write this book, but there are many, many others who do not have big offices but have given me their time and instruction. There is a symbiotic relationship between journalists and public relations agents, and I have had great help from Frankie Akute. He led me to two of my most important sources—Pamela Were and Anyara Papa. He also provided a reliable sounding board upon which I tested ideas. You do not go wrong listening to Frankie. Beryl Maritim is the other PR person I learned the most from. She patiently explained population health to me more than once and tolerated my slow learning curve like a generous teacher.

Pamela and Papa have already been mentioned here, but I also want to acknowledge the many others who feature significantly in my account. Kenneth Kisuya Malaba, Mustafa Ghulam, Edith Apondi Ogalo, Jane Chemon, Archie Shume, Joyce Oboi, Grace Bor, Judy M. Butu, Nyareso Mokaya, Ann Morogo, Dennis Munyoro, Judy Odiwa, Ann Jeptoo Tallam, Joel Chanda, Gideon Kemboi, Hillary Kiptoo, Joseph Binayo, Dolly Nyang'wera, Susan Rono, Brian Kipchumba Sang, Byrum Angote, Dominic Serem, Benjamin Andama, Cleophas Chesoli, Abraham Boit, Pamela Busieney, Donald Cheminingwa, Stephen Kiptoo, Nicolas Kisilu, Chris Mwaniki, John Okeyo, Beatrice Betty Obiero, Elisha Onyango Okeyo, Ebby Opisa, Elizabeth Nanyama, Judith Nandwa Lubanga, Marian Rotich, Margaret Fwamba, Faustin

Obbo Otin, Bernard Odkicipbo, Millicent Amolo, Judy Koech, Sampson Araka, Jane Omutsani, David Onyango, Benjamin Andama, Wilson Kipkirui Aruasa, Paul Ayuo, Adrian Gardner, Laura Ruhl, Sonak Pastakia, Wilson Nyandiko, Jeremiah Laktabai, Megan Miller, Julia Songok, Fredrick Asirwa Chite, Tim Mercer, Rajesh Vedanthan, James Lemons, Manu Chandaria, Patrick Loehrer Sr., Dave Matthews, Hal Campbell, Samwel Kimani, Kara K. Wools-Kalostian, Robert Rono, Agustine Miencha, Jessica Ruff, Matthew Turissini, Peninah Mshindi, and Leonard Otieno all helped me, often over and over.

And now I simply list the names of folks who helped me along the way as I wandered around Eldoret. Each deserves more, but I hope this reminds them of my gratitude. Geofrey Omondi, Megan Miller, Ron Pettigrew, Bornice Chepng'etich Biomndo, Chris Murphy, Peter Chiliswa, Sharon Chemtai, Miriam Barr, Victoria Eder, Talmage Bosin, Lukoye Atwoli, Debbie Ungar, Helen Wu Li, Francis Dagala, Beatrice Jakait, Rose Ayikukwei, Dino Martins, Shadrack Kirop, Alex Farris, Jessica Contrera, Katie Mettler, Sampson Boyo, David Plater, Mariam Kanyugo, Rehab Cheruiyot, Christine Chuani, Jess Gardner, Michael Scanlon, Gregory Schmidt, Mikey Clark, Caitlin Delong, Arnold Obungu, Nate DeLong, Michelle Kitsis, Julie Thompson, John Humphrey, Eunice Kamaara, Ian McIntosh, Jordan Huskins, Geren Stone, Christine Stone, Matt Strother, Terry Vick, Gail Vance, Karen Yoder, Myrta Pulliam, Tom Inui, Rakhi Karwa, Rompus Onyatch, Connie Keung, Elsie Rotich, Violet Naanyu Yebei, Peter Kussin, Jonathan Dick, Edward Liechty, Joseph Chacha, Constantine Mwanga, Max Waweru, Paul Oloo, Sammy Githuku, Jepchirchir Kiplagat, Emmanuel Koros, Richard Mibey, Matu Mguri, Tina Dan Tran, Lindsey Haskett, Naiomi Lundman, Imran Manji, Bryce McKey, Milkah Cheptinga Murugi, Deborah Hirt Neary, Patrick O'Meara, Neelima Navuluri, Dennis K. Sang, John Lawrence, Sara Fletcher, Han Sitters, Magdaline Chepkemoi, John Kibosia, Justus Wamukoya, Purity Korir, Joshua Kwonyike, Thomas Kipkurgat, Anne Nangulu, Charles Ochieng' Ong'ondo, Wycliffe Agela, Dunya Karama, Joseph Kimani Munyua, Daniel Lang'at, Henry Kerre Wakhungu, and Jerry Wagner.

Long ago my favorite journalism professor taught me that every good writer needs an editor. Because I am primarily a photojournalist, that surely goes double for me. My Fulbright supervisor and long-time friend Abraham Mulwo content edited my final draft in fall 2020. He helped me with several matters of local Kenyan culture that I would have been embarrassed by and fixed numerous other flaws. But mostly, he assured me that I could publish with confidence. He told me:

> I have read several books about Africa that are written by *mzungu* authors who often seem to interpret activities and contexts they are describing from a Western perspective. The common trend is to highlight how Western experts are out there saving helpless locals (almost similar to what we see in Hollywood movies). Your story is different. It is about individuals from across the world coming together to share ideas and expertise with local actors, and in the process learning from one another, while at the same time successfully tackling a health crisis. The end result is a model for managing chronic diseases that several countries are now seeking to replicate. I am particularly impressed by your ability to enable the various actors in your book to tell their own story about their interaction with the AMPATH program. By so doing, you have allowed the reader to see the story of AMPATH as it unfolds, and to interpret this story from their own perspective, rather than yours.

I was also encouraged and guided nicely by the folks working for the IU Press. Dr. Gary Dunham is the director of the press, but acted as my acquisitions editor because the pandemic had shrunk his staff by the time my manuscript and photos were delivered to him. He helped me stay on task with clear direction and calm encouragement. Carol McGillivray and Nancy Lightfoot assisted with the copyediting, and I marvel at their ability to find my typos, missing citations, and many style errors, but especially their willingness to ever so gently suggest how my prose could be a bit more clear, er, I mean, "clearer." Cyndy Brown created the index and alerted me to several typos in the proofreading stage that I would have been embarrassed by. Thank you editors, indexer, and proofreaders all.

And, maybe most important of all, I wish to thank my Moi University and Indiana University students who have learned about AMPATH and about collaboration between Kenyans and Hoosiers with me over the years. Through their eyes I have seen far more than I could have otherwise seen. Their reporting and our discussions have informed, encouraged, and inspired me.

NOTE ON LANGUAGE

SWAHILI AND ENGLISH ARE THE TWO official working languages of Kenya, although a total of sixty-eight languages are spoken in Kenya. This variety is a reflection of the country's diverse population, which includes most of the major ethnoracial and linguistic groups found in Africa (Greenberg 1970). Virtually all AMPATH employees speak English fluently, although all also speak Swahili and their local language, which, in the area AMPATH serves, is mostly Kalenjin, Luhya, Dholuo, and Gusii. My Swahili allows me to exchange greetings and pleasantries but little beyond that. All personal interviews and the online survey were conducted in English. Kenyans use British spellings and drop Swahili words into their conversations as if they were English. I provide translations for those few words in the narrative on first occasion only. I have used American English spellings and imperial units for distances (except in quotations) because the IU Press is American, even though this will read oddly to Kenyans. I have given the value of money in Kenyan shillings and then converted into US dollars. On first reference, I precede AMPATH employees with either Dr., Ms., Mr., Professor, or Dean as a way of acknowledging that all are worthy of respectful titles, regardless of academic degree.

ABBREVIATIONS

AIDS	acquired immunodeficiency syndrome
AMPATH	Academic Model Providing Access to Healthcare
AMPATH Plus	The USAID-funded portion of AMPATH focused exclusively on HIV/AIDS
AMRS	AMPATH Medical Record System
ART	antiretroviral therapy
ARVs	antiretroviral drugs
CCC	comprehensive care clinic
CDC	Centers for Disease Control and Prevention
CHV	community health volunteer
CHW	community health worker
COBES	community-based experience and service
FPI	Family Preservation Initiative
GESP	group empowerment service provider
GISHE	Group Integrated Savings for Health and Empowerment
HHI	HAART and Harvest Initiative
HIT	health information technology
HIV	human immunodeficiency virus
HTC	home testing and counseling

IRB	Institutional Review Board
IREC	Institutional Research and Ethics Committee
IU	Indiana University
IUPUI	Indiana University Purdue University Indianapolis
KNH	Kenyatta National Hospital
KSh	Kenyan shilling (approximately one shilling to one US cent)
LACE	Legal Aid Centre of Eldoret
LDL	low detectable level of the HIV virus
MOAQJSS	Michigan Organizational Assessment Questionnaire Job Satisfaction Subscale
MoE	Ministry of Education
MoH	Ministry of Health
MOU	memorandum of understanding
MTRH	Moi Teaching and Referral Hospital
MUCHS	Moi University College of Health Sciences
NCK	Nursing Council of Kenya
NHIF	National Hospital Insurance Fund
NIH	National Institutes of Health
NYU	New York University
OGW	Order of the Grand Warrior of Kenya
OVC	orphans and vulnerable children
PDA	personal digital assistant
PEPFAR	President's Emergency Plan for AIDS Relief
PJP	*Pneumocystis jirovecii* pneumonia
PMTCT	prevention of mother-to-child transmission of HIV
PrEP	pre-exposure prophylaxis
RFP	revolving fund pharmacy
RSPO	Research and Sponsored Projects Office
SIU	Southern Illinois University
STI	sexually transmitted infection
TB	tuberculosis
USAID	United States Agency for International Development
UT	University of Texas
WAMI	Work and Meaning Inventory
WHO	World Health Organization

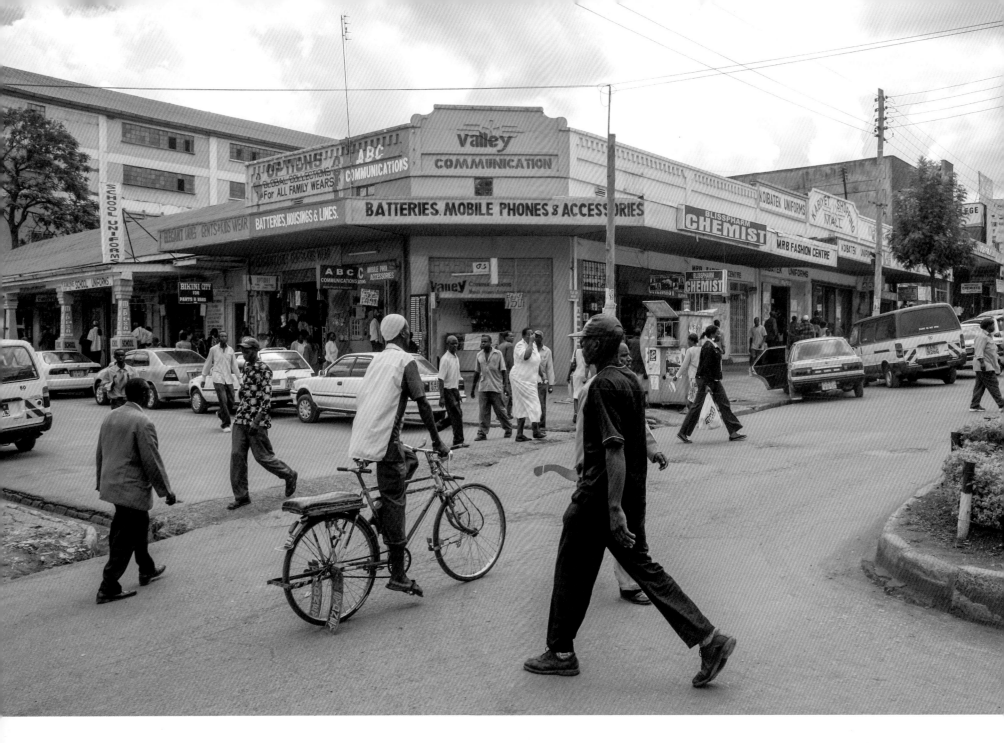

Pedestrians and a bicycle taxi driver move about downtown Eldoret near the roundabout at Oginga Odinga and Elijah Cheriyot streets, with a view of the Kabiyet Shopping Mall, in 2009.

PART ONE

INTRODUCTION

CHAPTER ONE

My African Experience

Human beings originated in Africa, and anthropology still marks the Great Rift Valley in the eastern portion of the continent as a likely location for the birthplace of *Homo sapiens*. Africa is our home. Most of us have been away a very long time, and some of us never left.

This is a story about both human beings who never left and human beings who recently returned. It is a story about Kenyans and Hoosiers. It is a story about providing healthcare through a partnership that motivates its staff to levels of excellence not common in the developing world. It is about economic and social development done right. It is about a partnership among doctors and nurses, pharmacists and clinicians, social workers and counselors, and deans and professors—all working together in a special collaborative relationship that has been providing community healthcare, medical training, and academic

research for more than thirty years. It is a sustainable development program that has been improving the lives of hundreds of thousands with little fanfare but fabulous results. The story of the Academic Model Providing Access to Healthcare (AMPATH) is known by far too few, and it is loved by all who have heard of and lived it. I'm not the first to share this story, and I won't be the last, but certainly no one can ever hear a good story too many times.

When I first visited East Africa in 2002, I was surprised by how much it felt like home—the place literally seemed designed to live in. I have heard this from others who love the Great Rift Valley, both the people who were born there and the people who visit. The weather is perfect. It gets hot, but not too hot. It gets cold, but not too cold. Some months have enough rain to make the rivers run fast. Other months do not, and the rivers flow slowly. The sun shines for twelve hours each day and then disappears for the other twelve. There is a moment every day when the sun is directly above your head and the earth is directly below your feet. It is a place of equilibrium where things change, but at the same time remain the same. A place where I am a stranger from a distant land but where everyone welcomes me as if I had just returned from a journey. Every time I visit, it feels like I belong, even though I was not born there and have no claim to it as my own. Perhaps it is the way that people greet you with a gentle handshake and the words *karibu sana* ("you are very welcome" in Swahili). Or that they are so quick to take you into their homes and share their food and live their lives with you. "You are family" comes surprisingly soon after the initial meeting. I feel at home even though I am clearly *mzungu*.

Mzungu, literally translated, means "someone who roams around aimlessly," but it is generally understood as "white foreigner." These definitions speak to the heart of the relationship between African and not African. Many white visitors today, like the European explorers of precolonial Africa, do indeed wander somewhat aimlessly, driving around game parks, visiting wild-animal orphanages, or perhaps building schools or latrines for villagers. They are welcomed, but their purpose is not often understood. This book is about Kenyans who welcomed *wazungu* (plural form) from Indiana (Hoosiers) and joined with them to create an understanding about how to provide quality healthcare to the people of Kenya.

In January 2019, my wife, Carol, and I left our home in Bloomington, Indiana, to spend a semester living as *wazungu* in Eldoret, Kenya. We are both white. I was on a sabbatical from Indiana University (IU) and had been awarded a Fulbright Scholar grant. Carol had just retired so she could join in the adventure. My project was to document the work of an amazing partnership between the

medical schools at IU and Moi University. In the 1990s, the two universities had joined with Kenya's Ministry of Health to build the country's second medical school and transform a district hospital into the country's second tertiary care facility.

Ten years later, during the first decade of the twenty-first century, that IU-Kenya Partnership mobilized an effort to end the HIV/AIDS epidemic then ravaging the country. Heroic efforts by Kenyans and North Americans working at AMPATH brought the epidemic under reasonable control by 2010. Many of the people who had led this effort were still working for AMPATH in the area's hospital and clinics in 2019, and I spent most of my days observing them as they cared for the people who depend upon the public health system. Each of these healthcare workers had been touched, in some way, by the epidemic at its height, and all still worked in an organization profoundly shaped by it. They had learned invaluable lessons from AMPATH's unique responses to HIV, and they were now applying those lessons to other diseases in distinctive ways. It was clear we had arrived at a time that everyone seemed to recognize as the end of one era and the beginning of another.

A Farewell Party for the IU House Family

On a beautiful Saturday in mid-March of 2019, Dr. Joe and Mrs. Sarah Ellen Mamlin started saying their good-byes. They had been leaders of AMPATH since before it was AMPATH, and they were going to retire for a second time and move back to Indiana. The farewell party was a relatively small gathering just up the hill from the house the Mamlins had called home since their return to a town they had first visited in 1989. In 2000, Joe had retired as the director of Wishard Memorial Hospital in Indianapolis,

and he and Sarah Ellen had decided to transition into their first retirement by serving as field directors in the IU-Kenya Partnership's operation in Eldoret for a year. They had arrived as the HIV/AIDS epidemic was decimating the country. Now, twenty years later, they were leaving at a time when HIV was being treated much like any other communicable disease. They came as *wazungu*, and as they left they were considered "honorary Kenyans" by everyone who knew them. They had been the longest of the long-term residents of a compound known as the IU House, a half-dozen buildings scattered throughout a small estate about two thousand feet up the river that formed the southern edge of the neighborhood. Their departure evoked great sadness and a bit of fear. Things would not be the same without the Mamlins, and everyone at IU House that day knew it.

Dr. Laura Ruhl, a former student of Joe's and now a senior leader of the organization he had helped found, had arranged for tents and tables, a disc jockey, and party decorations. The food was provided by the Sikh Union Club's restaurant, whose owner, Mr. Pritpal, chatted on the lawn with Mr. Yu, the owner of Siam Restaurant. The two of them had been feeding the Mamlins and their colleagues at the IU House for many years, but the Mamlins were much more than customers to them. Sarah Ellen's sister in Georgia had helped Yu's daughter attend university there. Joe had cared for Pritpal's relatives in the Moi Teaching and Referral Hospital. Every Wednesday was "cook's night off" at the IU House, and all residents—long and short term—had regularly eaten at Siam and Sikh Union, where the Mamlins sat with the owners. These old friends, Yu and Pritpal, were the only people who didn't live or work at the IU House. This was a family gathering, and they were most certainly part of the IU family, as were several North Americans from AMPATH-affiliated universities in other states, whom the locals nevertheless called Hoosiers.

Many at the party were wearing African-print dresses or shirts. Everyone was there. The *wazungu* were doctors, nurses, and pharmacists. Some had lived in Eldoret for a decade, some had been there for a few months, and still others had been spending their vacations working alongside Joe, Sarah Ellen, Laura, and the other long-term residents for many years. The staff were managers, accountants, guards, house cleaners, and maintenance workers. Some had worked for IU since the first house was leased back in the 1990s, and some had just started a few years back. Joe's longtime but now retired driver, Mr. David Onyango, was there too. He brought a plaque that said *"Hakuna Matata"* to give to the Mamlins. The party was part reunion and part intimate gathering of folks who had built lives together.

Dr. Adrian Gardner, the field director who had taken over from Joe seven years earlier, read his speech from a sheet of paper because, as he stated, "I know I won't get through this if I don't." He continued:

There really are no words that can capture the extraordinary impact you have had on this place, and on all of us. As Joe likes to say, the book will never be written. . . . You have been the matriarch and the patriarch of this family. You have been like parents to many of us, grandparents to our children, friends to us all. We have turned to you literally hundreds or thousands of times for advice and for help. You two, both individually, and even more so together, are the definition of grace, love, humility, and selflessness. You are responsible for this community, and we thank you for that. It will not be the same without you.

He got through it just fine, but not without dropping a tear at the end.

Next came Mr. Leonard Otieno, a guard who had spent hundreds of his night shifts in a small shed in front of the IU House while studying for a master's degree the Mamlins helped fund. Leonard read a speech on behalf of the entire staff: "You gave us all hope and taught us a lot through your actions daily. The gap, the void, is going to be chiasmic. We dread it, but we cannot avoid it, nor can we change it. Go and have a good rest. You have earned it. But please do remember us. You shall forever remain in our hearts." He also shed a tear before handing the microphone to Joe.

And then Joe, who does not welcome the limelight, gave a short speech with Sarah Ellen by his side. He started by protesting he had not prepared a speech and then pulled a few index cards from the pocket of his blue dress shirt. He said, "The greatest time of Sarah Ellen's and my life occurred after retirement. . . . We only work with two rules. You know them pretty well because we've all said them to each other . . . 'dream all night, and work all day.' Anybody dreaming without working? You're going nowhere. Anybody working without a dream? Where's that going to go? . . . I think this group is poised to do things that we never dreamed were possible. . . . As Sarah and I leave, we're better people because we were here."

As the two octogenarians went to the table to cut the cakes, they were flanked by the children of IU House. Laura Ruhl asked the crowd, "Cake song! Who knows the cake song?" Several of the Kenyans responded, "Kata kata. Kata cake kata. Kata tukule keki." Clapping and African ululation rang out. Ms. Peninah Asiimwe, the house cook, soon had the mic. She sang the cake song and led the staff women in a little dance. It was impromptu and joyous.

As the party wound down, everyone wanted a photo with the Mamlins—one last remembrance of people who had literally helped save the region from disaster. They knew very well that they had lived among true heroes and that their time with them was coming to an end. There would forever be the time when Joe Mamlin was with them and the time he no longer was.

How I Got to Eldoret

My sabbatical was not my first visit to Eldoret. I had first heard of AMPATH just weeks after joining the Indiana University School of Journalism in 2007. Dean Brad Hamm called me into his office to say that the IU School of Medicine in Indianapolis had asked him how our school might help his school increase awareness of the work they were doing in Africa. Brad knew I had worked in East Africa for years while on faculty at Southern Illinois University (SIU). I had led or helped with projects supported by the US Department of State's Office of Citizen Exchanges aimed at strengthening the ability of African journalists to report about the AIDS epidemic, which had been overwhelming the continent's healthcare system. My SIU colleagues and I had organized dozens of workshops in East Africa, and we had brought a few dozen East African journalists to the United States for still more training. I knew quite a bit about journalism and the epidemic in Ethiopia, Uganda, Tanzania, and Kenya, but I had never heard about AMPATH, and it seemed odd that I had not.

Brad said the IU School of Medicine had a program that was helping a medical school at Moi University in Eldoret, Kenya, provide testing for HIV, the virus that causes AIDS. They had also been treating HIV-positive people with antiretroviral drugs. I was curious. Associate Dean Bonnie Brownlee and I arranged a meeting on IU's Indianapolis campus with Mr. Fran Quigley, the partnership's director of operations, for the following month. Fran was also a freelance journalist, and I could relate to his passion for storytelling and his affection for Africa. I

had read a few articles he had written about the partnership for *NUVO*, the Indianapolis alternative newspaper, before we met, and I was excited to meet him. I would later learn that at the time we met, he was writing a book about the partnership that would provide the definitive history of what I would soon come to understand was an incredibly well-built and well-run operation.

There was talk of us going to Eldoret over winter break, but I suggested we might want to wait until spring break, since the Kenyan elections would be held in December. Sadly, those elections were followed by the worst intertribal violence the country had ever experienced. More than one thousand people died from the postelection violence, including around eighty children who were burned to death in a church just five miles outside Eldoret. I had read about this violence in the newspapers and lamented the fact that this sort of event is what most Americans know about Africa: violence, famine, poverty, and AIDS. But this means they do not know Africa. Many do not know where it is on a map or even that it is dozens of countries and not just a monolithic continent. They do not know that its landmass is three times bigger than the US, its population is nearly three times as large, and the history of its people is far more than three times as ancient.

We Americans are largely ignorant of Africa as our place of origin, and I, like most Hoosiers, did not know about AMPATH. I decided I needed to change that, and my idea was to take IU journalism students to Kenya so they could tell the stories of the people of Eldoret. I was a journalist by training and craft, and I had been teaching journalism for nearly two decades at that point. As a journalist, I had covered the start of the HIV epidemic in Indiana in the 1980s, and I had taught East African journalists how to cover the epidemic in the early 2000s through grants from the US Department of State. Now I wanted to teach students how to report about the tireless medical staff at AMPATH, who were saving lives at remarkable rates amid the worst pandemic since the Black Death of 1350.

In 2009, I was training journalists in Nairobi, Kenya's capital, and took a few days to visit Eldoret. I had arranged a meeting with Professor Wilphredian "Obi" Okumu-Bigambo, head of the communication department at Moi. Instead of a one-on-one meeting in his office, the whole faculty greeted me in the West Campus Faculty Parlor. Together, we talked about how we could collaborate and quickly came up with a plan: the next summer, I would bring a dozen IU journalism students to Eldoret, and Obi would select a dozen Moi students to join them.

During their coursework, these students formed twelve two-person reporting teams. Their interviews took them wherever AMPATH met clients: the villages, the farms, the slums, and the streets of Eldoret. My students learned from Obi's, and his learned from mine. We published thirty-six stories with photos to the IU School of Journalism's website, and several of the stories were published by the newspapers in Eldoret. We had used the AMPATH model. Ours was a partnership built on individual counterpart relationships.

And because AMPATH is all about sustained relationships, we taught the course again in 2011 and 2013 with one of Obi's junior faculty members, Professor Abraham Mulwo. The people our students reported about during those summer courses were mostly employees of the Ministry of Health (MoH) working as part of the AMPATH project and their patients and clients. My IU students were regularly surprised that their sources did not know that AMPATH was not entirely Kenyan. The partnership, started by a handful of Moi and IU professors twenty years earlier, was by that time a highly evolved organization of more than a thousand Kenyan healthcare workers who

looked like any other MoH professionals to their patients and clients. Few knew that the extraordinary care they were receiving had been nurtured by a pledge between a public university in Indianapolis and a public university in Eldoret to stay together for the long haul.

AMPATH's motto was and remains Leading with Care. Most international partnerships in medicine are exclusively research operations. AMPATH does conduct research, but its academic model argues that community healthcare must be the primary mission if sustainable and comprehensive population health is to be achieved. AM-PATH today is a partnership among the MTRH (Moi Teaching and Referral Hospital), Moi University College of Health Sciences (MUCHS), and a dozen North American university medical programs led by Indiana University. It is driven by the fundamental principal that strengthening a healthcare system "is built on the integrity of mutually beneficial and mutually respectful individual counterpart relationships between North Americans and Kenyans at all levels" (Mercer et al. 2018, 45). AMPATH's innovative approach is increasingly recognized as effective, and it was the brainchild of a relatively small group of medical academics who gave it life in a regional city in Kenya back in 1990.

To truly understand how the partnership plan launched three decades ago grew to a project that serves more than 600,000 people (180,000 of whom are HIV positive), one needs to talk with, observe, and learn from the extraordinary people who make up AMPATH today. They are medical specialists, including hospital administrators, general practice and specialty physicians, hospital nurses and home health aides, dentists, radiologists, therapists, pharmacists, nutritionists, and laboratory technicians, but they are also lawyers, social workers, counselors, software programmers, agriculturalists, farm laborers, janitors, and transport drivers. The range of occupations undertaken by people who work for AMPATH and are devoted to its mission is extraordinary because of the holistic approach of the partnership since its inception. AMPATH today cares for the whole person and the whole community. Exactly how that can evolve is evident in the partnership's history and its contemporary practice.

This chapter provides a glimpse into the extraordinary relationships that underpin and sustain one of the most successful North–South collaborations I know of and how I went about documenting the way Kenyans and their friends from North America put this holistic academic theory into practice every day. Fundamentally, this is a story about what it means to "lead with care," because that is the open secret of the collaboration's success.

Why Study AMPATH?

So why is the Academic Model Providing Access to Healthcare successful at sustaining long-term collaboration between Western universities from developed economies and a university in a rural part of the developing world?[1] A recent external analysis of the project by McIntosh and Kamaara argues that "this North–South partnership is uniquely placed to address the global public health crisis of HIV/AIDS while simultaneously providing a replicable model for success in Kenya and elsewhere" (McIntosh and Kamaara 2016, 256). I believe they are right.

Chapter 2 is a brief history of AMPATH that provides insight into how the relationship developed, but I do not think any recitation of dates and projects and name changes can adequately describe the heart of such an organization. AMPATH is not just an acronym. It is passion and love and devotion. It springs from the very souls of those who make it breathe so that it might give life to those it touches. It is the people of the Great Rift Valley working side by side with friends from North America.

1. I use *developing* / *developed world* terminology at the suggestion of the Associated Press Stylebook. For me, *developed* refers to economies that benefited economically from colonialism and *developing* refers to countries that are still recovering from foreign exploitation. I use *Third World* only to reference my earliest education in international development studies.

This is a book about what motivates the Kenyans who do the daily work of AMPATH, from nurses and doctors testing for sickle cell anemia and cervical cancer to counselors helping adolescents come to grips with learning they have been HIV positive since birth. It is about extension workers helping farmers raise dairy cows and microfinance officers instructing the mothers of a village about how to provide care to each other. Why do these employees work so hard for so little pay in such challenging conditions? What is it about AMPATH that inspires such loyalty and devotion to mission? I have talked with many doctors, administrators, and upper-level leaders at AMPATH over the years, and their dedication is extraordinary. Their successes are regularly written up in academic journals, celebrated during awards ceremonies, and acknowledged by university deans and ministry officials. I have read the articles, attended the ceremonies, and met the officials. There is no doubt that these leaders provide inspiration and guidance to the hundreds who work in less glamorous healthcare occupations, but they are not the "worker bees" who carry out AMPATH's mission.

During the summer classes I had taught years earlier, my journalism students were able to talk with the lower-level staffers and see the incredible work they did. I was envious of their experience. I wanted to see for myself the difference these unsung heroes were making in the lives of ordinary Kenyans every day, day after day, year after year. The AMPATH project is unique. It is so incredible and so inspiring that I believe it can only be explained by those staffers. Careful analyses by AMPATH professors, deans, and ministry officials provide impressive statistics and illuminate beautiful goals. But life is breathed into those diagrams and charts by hundreds and hundreds of medical personnel who have been educated and trained according to an ethos that was birthed three decades ago when earnest Hoosiers from the United States sat down

with an imaginative and innovative Kenyan who had a medical school to build. They had talked about partnership and friendship and the philosophy of *andū nio indo*, which, loosely translated from Kikuyu, means "wealth is people." Their shared belief that people have what they need inside them is what ultimately motivates the staff and fuels the work that provides health and happiness to the people of western Kenya.

And so dozens of times over the five months I was on sabbatical, I sat down with staffers and asked them to tell me what I needed to know. They explained to me, clearly and kindly, why they care, why they dare, and why they bear the burden of providing healthcare to the population the academic model addresses. I made documentary photographs of those same people and others as they went about their daily tasks. I drove down the red-dirt roads to the villages and farms where most of Africa lives. I sat in their clinics, shared tea with them around plastic tables, and patiently observed them as they comforted the sick and empowered the healthy. I was welcomed into their homes, and laughed with their spouses and children and friends. I had been given the chance to return to the place where human beings originated, and I reveled in the warm embrace. It is not enough to read about such dedication. One must see it—in person, as I have, or through photographs such as mine here.

How I Have Tried to Tell This Story

I have mentioned that I am white, and this begs the question of how I can possibly tell the story of Africans. The opportunity to try springs from my privilege. I was born in the developed world—the United States. My parents were not particularly wealthy by US standards, but we were fabulously rich by Kenyan standards of 1957. We lived in a democracy where education was free to all. My

parents encouraged my interests, and by their luck and their support, I became the first child in the family to earn a college degree. I worked as a newspaper journalist and eventually earned a doctorate in mass communication. I joined a university faculty, applied for some government grants, and began traveling the world to train journalists in developing countries.

It has been a charmed life. I married a wonderful woman, and we have two brilliant daughters. We lived in safe neighborhoods with good healthcare and plenty to eat. But for a month of every year, I managed to escape my bubble of privilege and travel to the other side of the planet where I could see how life was lived in the Third World that I had read about in college. My partner on those development grants, Dr. Jyotika Ramaprasad, was born in India and taught me countless lessons about how most of the world lived. She helped me see from a new perspective—still white and still "too tall," but from inside rather than outside. I am forever grateful for her teaching and remain a bit embarrassed that I was not a very quick study. I slowly came to understand that I was born of a tiny minority and that the majority was little known to me and little understood by my peers either. She and I trained dozens of journalists in India, Bangladesh, Nepal, Pakistan, Sri Lanka, Tanzania, Uganda, Ethiopia, and Kenya. I came to understand that, as their teacher, I was responsible not only for teaching them but also for learning from them.

Journalists tell other people's stories. If we listen carefully, observe diligently, and open our hearts, we are able to tell a story that fairly closely resembles what we heard and saw and felt. It is never perfect. It is never as complete as the story told to us, but if we try hard, it rings true to those who know nothing of the topic as well as those who know everything—audience and source.

The techniques I used to get the story close to right are described in chapter 9, "Methodology." For now, suffice it to say that with every source I met, I explained why I was asking them questions and taking their photos. I explained who I was and what had brought me to them. I asked them to share their story with me. I pledged to get it as right as I could. I recorded their voices, their faces, and their places. I wrote things down in notebooks purchased from the Naivas Supermarket with pens I had pilfered from my hotel room at the Nairobi Serena. I took hundreds of photos at every event or meeting, edited them down to a couple dozen I thought told the story, and then loaded them onto a tablet so I could return and ask the folks in the pictures if I had gotten it right. I told them I did not want to be the *mzungu* whose photos embarrassed them. I begged them to tell me if anything was wrong. If they did, I dropped the image from consideration. After writing up a chapter, I emailed it to the folks I quoted to make sure my colleague and Moi University graduate student, Mr. Geoffrey Omondi, had accurately transcribed their words from the tape recordings I had made. Geoffrey also reviewed much of my work and let me know how I was doing as I collected the interviews and photos for the book. I did all I could think of to check my privilege and make sure my perspective was as close to that of my subjects as I could get.

It was not a perfect method. I would have liked to have had a Kenyan partner with me every minute. Geoffrey would have made a great partner. He is smart and observant and as dedicated as anyone I have ever met. But he had to teach and tutor and help run a university. My friend and faculty supervisor, Abraham Mulwo, would have been an excellent partner. Like his student Geoffrey, he is smart and organized, and he is also an accomplished researcher. But he had a university department and a government

commission to run. My friend Mr. Frankie Akute, the public relations officer I had sent my students to a decade earlier, would have made a great partner, but he had a full-time job in MTRH corporate communications and a master's degree to complete. No one was on sabbatical but me. So I took as much time from each of these friends as I dared and listened for the slightest hint of disapproval or unhappiness from them about how I was doing my research. It may be that they were exceedingly kind, because they certainly are. But not once did they tell me I was off track. They seemed to think I had the story right. They are my confidence.

And now you are my confidence. If you are not Kenyan and there's something you think I have wrong here, please tell me and I'll try to do better in the future. But if you are Kenyan and I have something wrong, please forgive me. It is my fault alone. My friends and sources all helped me understand as best they could. They were always patient with me. They took time to meet with me, respond to my WhatsApp messages, read drafts of this manuscript, and study my photos. They did everything I asked of them. If this book comes close to telling their story, it is because they were so very good at telling it to me in the first place. And that—their kindness—has been my greatest privilege of all.

How to Read These Stories

The story of AMPATH is literally hundreds of thousands of stories. Most are lived by ordinary Kenyans who become ill, visit a dispensary or clinic, get treated, and return to their home a bit healthier. Some are lived by extraordinary Kenyans who become educated, join a medical staff, treat patients, and return to their homes proud of having helped others. Some stories are more dramatic than others. And some are more enlightening in that they touch on what makes AMPATH unique and innovative.

I have told stories of both types in this book. Read them in any order that appeals to you. Though there is some advantage to reading them in order, I have tried to make each stand on its own. If you want to understand the history that delivered me to 2019, when I finally had the chance to observe AMPATH in action, read chapter 2, "History and AMPATH." I argue that the reason that AM-PATH workers are so devoted to the mission traces back to the history of colonialism in Kenya and the struggle to build a nation following a cruel invasion from Europe. I describe a bit about what organizational behavior research tells us about work motivation, so the reader can better understand what the Kenyans I listened to for five months were telling me. Chapter 3, "AMPATH Re-envisioned," describes how AMPATH transitioned itself from an organization confronting the HIV/AIDS health emergency during the millennium's first decade into a rebranded operation working to move Kenya toward a new, comprehensive system improving the health of every member of society through population health.

Chapters 4 through 7 are stories about the "worker bees"—the people who work at the community level to screen patients, train community volunteers, educate farmers, counsel adolescents, and generally do the work that allows the leaders to claim success in their research reports. This list is even less exhaustive than the leaders' list. There are more than 1,500 workers on the AMPATH payroll and thousands more who volunteer, participate, and benefit from programs run by the organization. I started by talking with the folks in public relations and corporate communication at AMPATH and the MTRH: Frankie Akute, Ms. Beryl Maritim, Ms. Sharon Chemtai, and Mr. Daniel Lang'at. I asked them what the most

the early 2010s. But I worried the stories I had collected might not truly represent AMPATH as a whole. My perspective is imperfect. I wanted a way to ensure that what I saw firsthand was roughly similar to the general attitude of all AMPATH employees. To take the pulse of AMPATH—to gain a sense of how satisfied staffers were with their jobs, how motivated they were to do the hard work, and whether they saw their work as meaning-ful as the folks I observed did—I conducted a survey of all 1,500 workers. Their responses form another sort of story bolstered with statistics and inferences. It may not appeal to all readers, but it provides a statistically reliable bit of evidence for those who may be skeptical of claims of great success made by administrators of grand projects and wonder what the people on the ground actually think. In chapter 9, I explain the methods I used to tell the stories presented in chapters 4 through 8, but I concentrate on how I conducted the survey using emailed invitations and a Google form on the internet. In chapter 10, I describe the findings from the survey and argue for their statistical reliability and practical validity.

Following all of the extraordinary stories from worker bees and their leaders and the presentation of social sci-entific measurement of the attitudes of all AMPATH workers, in chapter 11 I attempt a conclusion. It is the last chapter because if you do not make it that far, you will have missed only the least important story. However, my friends at AMPATH have told me my conclusion is pretty close to the truth. Trust them, just as I did.

innovative portions of AMPATH were and they told me about (1) population health and economic empower-ment, (2) private-public partnerships, (3) chronic disease management, and (4) Rafiki, a comprehensive care clinic for youths. There were certainly other innovative projects I could have included, but if you read these four chapters and listen to what the workers say about themselves, you should come away with a sense of how motivated these staffers are and how the success of their programs inspires them to do the work of building a better healthcare system for the region.

Chapter 8 is composed of eleven stories about the leadership. These folks head institutions, projects, and ini-tiatives. They have advanced degrees in medicine, phar-macology, and public health. They publish and maintain reputations in their professional circles. You cannot un-derstand AMPATH without knowing something about these eleven people I was fortunate to interview and pho-tograph while in Eldoret. But there is at least one leader I should have interviewed and did not. The list is not ex-haustive. By the time this book is published or you read it, one or more of these leaders may have moved on to a new position of authority and a new leader may have taken his or her place. But reading what these eleven leaders have to say provides relatively solid insight into the philosophy that drives AMPATH's success.

The leaders and the worker bees told me the incredible stories that seemed to match what I had read on AM-PATH's website and sounded so very similar to the re-porting my students had done about the organization in

CHAPTER TWO

History and AMPATH

AMPATH has a clear and obvious beginning, but that beginning is embedded in a complex history of foreign intervention in Africa. In 1988, Moi University School of Medicine Dean Haroun Mengech hosted a small group of faculty members from a medical school in Indiana. That was the beginning of the partnership, no doubt, but the relationships formed during that visit were preceded by decades of less than noble interactions between people who had lived between Mount Kenya and Lake Victoria and people who had come from beyond the shores of Africa. The medical doctors from Indianapolis seemed kind, but there was a history of Western medical practice in the Great Rift Valley that did not augur well for a trusting relationship.

Melissa Graboyes (2014) notes that Western medicine arrived in Africa alongside European explorers in the mid-1800s. She reminds us that the history of medical research in East Africa is fraught with exploitation—part and parcel of colonial manipulation and oppression. Western medical doctors began with an assumption that Africa was a source of data, a fertile testing ground, and a birthplace of discoveries (379). Early efforts regularly blended ostensibly charitable medical interventions with medical research and public health practices that too often involved human experimentation. East Africans were the human material necessary for research projects focused on malaria, trypanosomiasis (sleeping sickness), leprosy, onchocerciasis (river blindness), schistosomiasis (bilharzia), and lymphatic filariasis (elephantiasis), among other tropical illnesses. To protect themselves from these maladies, Europeans experimented on Africans. As vaccines, prophylaxes, and treatments were developed, the

ability of the Europeans to exploit the natural resources and human labor of the continent was enhanced. Africans benefited somewhat from these discoveries but certainly did not participate in the research as equal partners or even in most cases as willing subjects. Because medical research was regularly blurred with treatment, these encounters frequently created misunderstanding and skepticism. As was sadly common practice in the developing world, researchers often willfully misled people about the goals, outcomes, and accompanying risks of participation and even coerced people to obtain blood and other samples needed for experimentation. According to Graboyes, "These past encounters with medical research shape modern East Africans' interactions with, and understandings of, biomedicine" (380).

Kenyans' interaction with Western medicine, like their interconnection with the colonial structures that supported the healthcare system, was far more nuanced than many imagine. Historian George Ndège (2001) warns against a too-common misconception that Africans had been powerless in shaping colonial medical policy and colonial rulers were all powerful in shaping Kenya's healthcare system. He argues that "beneath the strands of tension and conflict there also existed a world of compromise, accommodation, and coexistence between African and Western biomedical practices" (xii). Kenyans were trained as clinicians, nurses, and other medical workers, but they were few in number, and they worked within a system designed to serve the needs of an occupying power. According to Ndège, "At independence in 1963, Kenya's health care system reflected its long colonial history. The health care system was elitist in its orientation, curative in its emphasis, uneven in its geographical distribution, and fragmented into two sectors, private and public/ government. The efforts of the transitional years, 1960 to

1965, were halting and uncertain as the postcolonial state sought to assert its authority over the key sectors: the economy, health, and education" (134). Colonial hospitals and research institutes became the responsibility of the new government, and many fell into disarray as British researchers and administrators returned to Europe rather than conform to Africanization policies. There were simply too few Kenyans trained to conduct research, and government efforts were focused on educating physicians who could provide primary healthcare to the population, not on funding research or programs of preventative medicine. Unfortunately, the historical emphasis on research and British university structures had also left the country with Kenyan professors who were insufficiently prepared to educate a new cadre of doctors and administrators to care for the millions of newly minted citizens. The Kenyan government needed to educate and deploy substantial numbers of doctors, nurses, and medical technicians into a healthcare system suffering from the exodus of the colonial medical expertise.

They had considerable success, much of it under the general effort of *harambee* ("all pull together" in Swahili), the Kenyan tradition of community self-help, bolstered by government funding directly to facility construction projects in underserved areas, including the rural areas surrounding Eldoret. Between 1963 and 1992, the number of hospitals, health centers, and dispensaries more than quadrupled. Medical training was centered at Kenyatta Hospital in Nairobi, the national referral hospital, which from 1970 doubled as a teaching hospital for the country's sole medical school at the University of Nairobi. The results are striking. Over that three-decade period, the average life span of a Kenyan went from forty to sixty years, infant mortality was cut in half, the number of doctors increased from 339 to 3,550, and the number of hospital

beds increased from 6,708 to more than 34,000. Kenya made great strides in developing a healthcare system serving Kenyans in a very short time (Republic of Kenya 1994, 119).

It was just twenty-five years after independence when the Hoosiers arrived in Eldoret. Kenyans remained leery of foreign expertise and were proud of the progress they had made in educating their medical personnel. They had built a system that was doing a far better job of providing healthcare to the general population than a generation earlier. They were not looking for help from foreigners. But the four doctors from Indianapolis who set off in November 1988 on a three-week world tour were looking for an international partner for the Indiana University School of Medicine, not a subject for their research. Drs. Bob Einterz, Joe Mamlin, Charlie Kelley, and Dave Van Reken were drawn to Eldoret, Kenya, not only because of its considerable need for medical care but especially because of the vision expressed by Mengech who had only recently been named dean of a yet-to-be established second medical school in Kenya. Mengech was on the lookout for partners.

Mengech had long been a critic of the old British lecture system for medical education that persisted after independence at the University of Nairobi's medical school in the nation's capital. In 1981, Kenyan president Daniel arap Moi appointed Canadian scholar Dr. Colin Mackay to head a commission to prepare plans for restructuring the country's higher education system and establishing a second national university. The several fundamental educational reforms recommended included ending the British examination system and requiring that bachelor's degrees consist of four years of university education. These reforms were in effect when Moi University in Eldoret was chartered in 1984. And because the commission's critiques

of the country's medical education system echoed those of Mengech, he was asked to head the new medical school. He was determined to build the school's curriculum around the broad, community-based service model he had championed throughout his professional career.

In 1985, just as the four Hoosier doctors would do three years later, Mengech traveled the world to visit medical schools with community-based curricula, including McMaster University in Canada and the University of Maastricht in the Netherlands. He determined that a community-based experience and service (COBES) program would be at the core of the new school's educational approach. Clinical experience would be emphasized as a way to connect textbook lessons with practice. This was radical thinking in Kenya at the time, and while Mengech had the support of the MoH, his medical colleagues in Nairobi were skeptical.

Bob and Joe had experienced similar reactions to their ideas about community-based education, but both knew from their own experience in the developing world that getting out of the clinic and meeting people where they lived—delivering health prevention and promoting care in the home and community spaces—were key to addressing the problems facing rural Africa.

While Mengech was searching the world for his school's educational model, Bob, fresh out of the IU School of Medicine, was working in Haiti, providing medical care without benefit of consistent supplies of medicines, electricity, or even water. He nevertheless strove to provide holistic care to his village. He learned firsthand about a physician's role in the community, the role of economics and culture in healthcare, and the importance of women in development.

"These were things not covered in med school, and they hit me in the face in rural Haiti," Bob recalled

(Quigley 2009, 23). After a year in Haiti, he returned to the IU School of Medicine in Indianapolis and began working to create opportunities for young doctors who wanted international experiences. His boss in the school's Division of General Internal Medicine was Joe Mamlin, who had learned similar lessons about community healthcare during his time spent in Afghanistan two decades earlier.

In 1965, Joe had spent two years in Jalalabad, Afghanistan, with the Peace Corps trying to help start a medical school. He had also faced shortages of everything: drugs, X-rays, blood, and equipment. And although he managed to persuade friends back in Indiana to donate needed materials, he left the country without having achieved the long-term solution he had hoped for. His focus on healthcare delivery had been thwarted by his local partner organization's inability to supply the basics. The Afghans earnestly desired to collaborate but lacked the resources required for effective partnership. Upon returning to Indianapolis, Joe worked to connect his IU school with the school in Afghanistan in a long-term relationship to provide community healthcare, but he was unable to do so. The idea was ahead of its time. But he had learned lasting lessons about the power of collaboration between partners that approached each other with mutual respect and focused on the provision of care rather than just research. The lessons these two doctors had learned in Haiti and Afghanistan informed their decision to seek an international partner. Their colleagues, Charlie Kelley and Dave Van Reken, had also spent time working in the developing world. Charlie had treated patients and taught in Afghanistan, and Dave had been a missionary in Liberia. They too saw the need for partnership focused on the practical problems of healthcare, and they believed a major medical school like IU's could prove instrumental in building medical capacity abroad.

The IU-Kenya Partnership

That initial meeting of Mengech, Bob, Joe, Charlie, and Dave in Eldoret in 1988 was the beginning of a long and sustained relationship between two medical schools that were about as different as could be. IU's school was more than eighty years old, and Moi's was just starting up. Interestingly, the IU School of Medicine was founded in 1903—the same year the first white Afrikaners from South Africa arrived in Eldoret to set up a massive farming operation on land previously inhabited by the Nandi people. The Nandi still live in the area and today use the services of AMPATH. But the years between that first European contact and the day Hoosiers and Kenyans came together on the high plateau of the Great Rift Valley to collaborate on community-based medicine produced two very different histories.

At the start of the twentieth century, Indiana was transitioning from an agricultural to an industrial economy with Indianapolis as the center of production (Phillips 1968). Nearly 170,000 people lived in the state's capital city, and the value of goods manufactured in the city was approximately sixty-nine million dollars annually (Geib 1981). Four major railways passed through Indianapolis's Union Station. The city was home to major meatpacking, grain-milling, vegetable-canning, and automobile-manufacturing plants, as well as banking and insurance companies (Esarey 1924). Demand for industrial labor encouraged new migration to the city from Indiana's rural areas. After World War I, it also drew large numbers of African Americans from the American South as well as English, Irish, German, Hungarian, Italian, and Greek immigrants from overseas. Indianapolis's schools were not segregated until 1927, when, with the rise of the Ku Klux Klan in the state, a Blacks-only high school was established despite

opposition from the African American community. The Klan's influence on state governance was considerable during the postwar era but was effectively ended during the 1930s after a series of scandals involving the governor and other members of the Klan. School segregation was outlawed in 1948. Indianapolis's population was, by then, about 15 percent African American.

The post–World War II period in Indianapolis saw further growth in industrial output and significant increases in the higher education sector. The city was home to major medical trauma centers, including Methodist Hospital (one of the largest private hospitals in the country) and several smaller hospitals. Over the years, the IU School of Medicine operated out of several buildings that eventually became known as the Indiana University Medical Center. Both Indiana University and Purdue University operated branch campuses that merged into Indiana University–Purdue University Indianapolis (IUPUI) in 1967. Today, Indianapolis has a population of 864,000, about 27 percent African American, within a metropolitan area of about 2 million with a per capita income of $31,186.

At the start of the twentieth century, in what was then the western region of the British East Africa Protectorate, the Nandi people were in the final throes of a decade-long war of attrition against the encroaching British Empire (Parsons 2012). The British had completed a railway from the Indian Ocean port of Mombasa to Lake Victoria in 1901, enhancing their ability to bring native lands under the Crown's control. Although skillfully led by the Nandi *orkoiyot* (primary spiritual and military leader) Koitalel arap Samoei, the local people lost the fight in 1905 after more than six hundred of their warriors were killed by King's African Rifles troops under the command of Colonel Richard Meinertzhagen. Under the terms of the peace settlement, the Nandi surrendered large sections of territory to the Uganda Railway. Just three years before Meinertzhagen's victory, the first white settlers, the Van Breda brothers, had come up from South Africa after having been displaced by the Anglo-Boer War fought between the British Empire and two Boer states in South Africa. By 1908 the brothers were joined by another forty Afrikaner families who settled the new town side by side with British colonials.

An extension of the Uganda Railway reached the European settlement of Eldoret in 1924. Goods could be imported cheaply, and farm produce could be transported out at competitive rates, leading to considerable growth in commercial output and population, including many immigrants from India who had come to Kenya as railway construction workers. The Afrikaners largely controlled agricultural output while the British controlled most of the commerce and industrial output, including milling and textiles. The Indians ran the shops, and the Africans served mostly as manual laborers. The town remained oddly divided between the two groups of white settlers until independence. During the 1950s, the town was literally divided along the main street—Afrikaners on the north and the British on the south. The former took their children to Highland School (now Moi Girls High School) and the latter to Hill School (still the Hill School).

After independence on December 12, 1963, substantial proportions of the Afrikaans and British populations left the area. Whites who agreed to take up Kenyan citizenship stayed, and most continued to operate large farms in rural areas like Eldoret. Indian descendants of those who had built the railways also took up citizenship in the new country. The schools the colonial governments had built came under the control of the new Ministry of Education (MoE), and faculty in Eldoret were soon teaching children who were mostly Black and brown and just a few who were white. The colonial hospital that had been established in 1916 with a bed capacity of sixty was reestablished as a district hospital under the MoH. The Kenyan government instituted a national healthcare system that quadrupled the number of healthcare facilities by 1985. Life expectancy increased from forty-eight to fifty-nine years by the mid-1980s, and child survival rates also improved dramatically (Yamin and Maleche 2017). Several private and charity hospitals were eventually established in Eldoret, including Eldoret Hospital, Mediheal Hospital, and Elgon View Hospital. The largest government facility today is the Moi Teaching and Referral Hospital (MTRH), one of only two national-level, tertiary care hospitals in the country.

About three hundred thousand people live in Eldoret, and the per capita GDP is probably a bit lower than the national average of $3,500. Nearly everyone in town is Black or brown except the Hoosiers, though several of them are also Black or brown. Tourism, while big business for Kenya, is quite limited. The city is the regional hub for the vast agricultural area around it. There is some manufacturing (mostly textiles), perhaps four dozen banks, and a range of higher educational institutions, including four technical and vocational institutes, six branch campuses of national universities, and the main campuses of two national universities, with Moi University being the largest in the area and the third largest university in Kenya. It was chartered in 1984 and is now a comprehensive university with more than fifty-seven thousand students pursuing undergraduate or graduate degrees in professional schools in business, engineering, law, and medicine and roughly a dozen doctoral programs.

Moi University enrolled its first medical class of forty students in 1990. Bob Einterz became the first IU faculty physician to spend a full year in Eldoret working as a field director of the collaboration then known as the IU-Kenya Partnership. In what was to be a regular rotation of "team leaders," Bob worked alongside the dozen newly hired faculty members at Moi's medical school. Together, they cared for Kenyan patients, conducted health research, and taught both Kenyan and American medical students. Six IU medical students and residents spent time in Eldoret that first year, and six Kenyan students spent time in Indianapolis. Soon, exchange programs were shuttling students and faculty back and forth between Eldoret and Indianapolis on a regular and recurring basis. Many of the medical staff at IU's medical facilities were also spending their vacations and leaves at MTRH, learning and teaching on the hospital's wards. Moi University faculty members earned fellowships that allowed them to learn, teach, and conduct research in Indianapolis. The exchanges provided lessons and experiences that enriched both medical and cultural learning and deepened the personal relationships between the Kenyan and Hoosier physicians devoted to the mission.

The HIV/AIDS Epidemic

The growing partnership between Moi and IU would soon be tested in dramatic fashion, however. President Moi could not have foreseen that at about the same time his Mackay Commission was proposing a dramatic restructuring of Kenya's medical education system, researchers in the United States were discovering a virus that would have devastating consequences for his country, and he could not have imagined that his proposed second medical school would play such a huge role in his nation's response to the epidemic then blooming in sub-Saharan Africa.

The reported history of HIV/AIDS began in 1981 when the Centers for Disease Control and Prevention

(CDC) in Atlanta reported described cases of *Pneumocystis* pneumonia in previously healthy gay men in Los Angeles. It was the first official reporting of what would soon be known as the AIDS epidemic. The CDC released the first case definition for AIDS the following year, and by 1984, HIV (human immunodeficiency virus) had been determined as the cause of AIDS and the first case in Kenya had been identified. By end of the next year, every region in the world had reported at least one case of AIDS, but the epicenter still seemed to be in the United States—not Africa.

We now know that HIV did not debut in the United States. It had been present in Africa since at least the 1920s, and by the 1970s, medical facilities in Uganda had observed cases of "slim disease" in the villages along Lake Victoria, just a couple hundred miles from Eldoret. Perfectly healthy fishermen would lose weight rapidly and die. But slim disease seemed unrelated to the AIDS outbreak among gay men in America and Europe. Slim was occurring predominantly in the heterosexually promiscuous population of women and men that fished the lake. They were dying of chronic diarrhea rather than Kaposi's sarcoma or other rare cancers associated with AIDS in America and Europe. But slim disease was in fact HIV, and the virus had been killing people in Africa for decades (Serwadda et al. 1985).

The pathological features of HIV/AIDS are unlike most other diseases. The early symptoms are easily overlooked because they are generally quite mild: fever, sore throat, and headache. They are easily dismissed as the flu or common cold. Even the most severe reactions during this "acute" stage recede after a week or two, when the virus passes into a latency period. Latency is largely asymptomatic. The virus replicates and begins to weaken the immune system, but a person at this stage does not feel or look sick. They can easily transmit the virus to others, though, and the stage typically lasts a decade before the immune system is weakened to the point that opportunistic infections kill the host. In regions where healthcare was minimal and life expectancy relatively short, people died of the virus without much notice because the disease that actually killed them was fairly common, like malaria or tuberculosis. Even a rare illness like *Pneumocystis jirovecii* pneumonia (PJP) was probably most often misdiagnosed as one of the more common forms of pneumonia. (PJP is the most common opportunistic infection found in HIV-positive people.) There is little doubt that AIDS had been in the area for a very long time, but the impact was small, and the effect went unnoticed in a region where diarrheal infection and lower respiratory infections were common and deadly.

That would change in the 1990s. During the first decade of the partnership, the main academic focus was on clinical education. Students and faculty members worked the hospital wards, learning and teaching. Reliable and cost-effective tests for HIV were increasingly available, and the doctors at the MTRH were confirming alarming increases in the number of people with the virus. The government of neighboring Uganda had dramatically reversed its country's HIV prevalence rate (the portion of the population with HIV) using a campaign of behavioral change that stressed abstinence, faithfulness, and condom usage, but Kenya's national leadership had resisted acknowledging the epidemic. The IU-Kenya Partnership had made great strides during its first decade. It had negotiated cultural differences and overcome financial constraints. It had trained hundreds of Kenyans and Americans who provided care in both the urban hospital and a growing number of rural clinics started by the ministry. But it could not imagine what lurked ahead.

IU's Joe Mamlin was the partnership's field director in 1992 and 1993, and he was encouraged by how quickly the relationship had grown and how substantial the partnership had become in such a short time. Upon his return to the United States, he continued to work with his colleagues in Indiana and Kenya on the project. Together, they enlarged the donor network and expanded community healthcare operations in the region. But those who followed Joe to Eldoret were increasingly dismayed by the impact of the HIV epidemic on the health of the region. At the decade's end, IU internist Dr. John Sidle returned from a stint as field director completely devastated by the daily ordeal of watching his AIDS patients die and frustrated by his inability to prescribe newly developed drugs that colleagues in Indiana were using to treat HIV. Though he had been successful on many other fronts, John left Kenya depressed and discouraged by the suffering and loss of life in Kenya due to HIV. Meanwhile, Joe had decided that another round as field director would provide a nice transition to retirement, so in 2000 he and his wife, Sarah Ellen, returned to Eldoret for another two-year stay.

Like John, Joe was shocked by the conditions on the wards at the MTRH. A decade earlier, about eighty people, mostly elderly, died in the hospital every year. Now, more than eighty people were dying every month, and they were mostly young people in the prime of life. Unlike most viruses, HIV does not so much affect the weak and old but instead kills young adults who are raising families and building careers. During the year before most patients entered the MTRH's recently created AIDS wards, they were probably working hard, caring for their children, tending their gardens, and contributing to the country's expanding economy. By the time HIV patients arrived at the ward, there was little the medical staff could do but treat the opportunistic infections they knew would soon kill their patients. The outlook was bleak. A few weeks after the Mamlins arrived, Andrew Natsios, the chief of the US Agency for International Development (USAID), said

it was impossible to provide antiretroviral drugs to the millions of Africans with HIV. The cost was too high, and the medical infrastructure was insufficiently developed to manage the lifelong treatment regime. He famously said that many Africans "don't know what Western time is," implying they would be unable to adhere to the strict dosing requirements (Herbert 2001). Indeed, the global health consensus at the time was that a haphazard application of the new drugs would actually worsen the pandemic by creating drug-resistant strains of the quickly mutating virus. Prevention was to be the only response. A positive HIV test would remain a death sentence in Africa.

Doctors do not accept such prognoses easily. Joe quickly concluded that the partnership could not continue as before. The AIDS epidemic was too great a challenge to be ignored, and he had no intention of standing by, watching his patients die. The patient who caused Joe to take this defiant stand was Mr. Daniel Ochieng.

Ochieng had lost a third of his body weight and was just seventy-two pounds when Joe recognized him as one of the Moi medical students. Ochieng had been moved from the medical student dormitory across the street in a wheelchair and deposited on an AIDS ward beside dozens of others who awaited their fate. Joe had made the rounds of the ward many times and knew it should not matter that Ochieng was a medical student. The virus in him was the same as in the others on the ward. But of course, it did matter. Ochieng was his student. Joe wanted him to be the first patient treated for HIV by the partnership, and he wanted to change the way the partnership addressed community healthcare. He began writing letters to Bob and his colleagues in Indiana, imploring them to find a way to treat HIV patients in Eldoret. Within two weeks, Dr. Craig Brater, IU School of Medicine's dean, agreed to send $10,000 to Kenya to provide for a year and a half of treatment for Ochieng. Almost immediately, the antiretroviral drugs delivered the "Lazarus effect" in Ochieng, an almost immediate and quite dramatic improvement in health indicators. The Lazarus effect was by then well known in the United States but had not yet been seen in the MTRH. Ochieng began to gain weight, resist infections, and recover his health quickly. After six weeks, he walked off the ward with vigor. He was the first AIDS patient at MTRH to have done so. Ochieng's recovery provided hope to the hospital's physicians and other medical workers that the epidemic could be defeated, and it inspired physicians at IU in Indiana to locate additional resources for the fight. The IU-Kenya Partnership was on the brink of becoming AMPATH—the Academic Model for the Prevention and Treatment of HIV/AIDS.

The Academic Model for the Prevention and Treatment of HIV/AIDS

AMPATH started in a small room in the MTRH where Joe began seeing additional HIV patients and treating them with donated drugs. One Moi physician who referred patients to the new clinic was Dr. Sylvester Kimaiyo. His sister Roselyn had died of AIDS four years earlier, and he was about to depart for Indiana on a year-long fellowship where he would study HIV drugs and treatment methods. On his return to Eldoret in 2002, he joined Joe in his HIV clinic and soon opened one of his own, becoming one of the first African physicians to routinely provide treatment for HIV/AIDS.

The first big grant to support the AMPATH initiative came in 2001 from a coalition of foundations that would fund HIV treatment for HIV-positive mothers about to deliver babies. The goal was to treat one thousand Kenyans for life. Kimaiyo soon joined AMPATH and was followed by community leaders who advocated for condom use, responsible sex practices, and testing. By the end of

the next year, AMPATH was operating HIV/AIDS clinics at the MTRH and at four rural health centers where altogether about eight hundred HIV-positive patients were receiving antiretroviral drugs (ARVs). By 2003, more than 80 percent of new mothers treated at the MTRH were agreeing to be tested, and surveys showed that the deadly myths about HIV were fading away. The stigma that HIV was somehow reserved for those who were promiscuous or otherwise immoral was being defeated by dozens of brave women whose lives had been saved by the drug treatment and who were declaring to those in their villages that HIV was a virus and not a sin.

Soon, AMPATH was being identified by HIV/AIDS organizations as a "best practice" model for treatment in Africa. The growth and success of the budding organization was based in the environment of trust and mutual respect established through the IU-Kenya Partnership. As a result of the work done in the 1990s, the new project had full support and integration with the government health system and had access to those facilities in the region. AMPATH would be run efficiently because the partnership had already been running efficiently.

Administering a lifelong medical treatment regime as development aid is very different from providing food or clean water or even agricultural assistance. Patients must be educated about drug dosing and regularly monitored for compliance and drug resistance. Sloppy administration could lead to widespread resistance and thereby compound an already dire situation. Poor compliance by patients could also contribute to drug resistance, so a reliable healthcare system was essential to overcome these reasonable threats. AMPATH was able to provide both the quality of care required and the drugs needed. They were also able to collect and store patient records in a computer system—the AMPATH Medical Record System. On average their patients proved to actually be better at taking their pills than similarly treated patients in the United States. The care and data provided by AMPATH's staff were reversing the tide of skepticism, and the drugs donated by foundations back in the United States were letting them reverse the tide of infection. The next big break was a $500,000 grant from the Purple Foundation of Canada in late 2002. The request for funding had been titled "A Bridge of Hope," and it allowed AMPATH to expand its treatment program from hundreds to thousands of clients. Later that year, AMPATH was given additional reason to hope that they would soon be on the other side of that bridge.

During his January State of the Union address in 2003, US president George W. Bush announced that because of generic forms being manufactured in Brazil and Argentina, the cost of HIV drugs had dropped low enough that he could propose the President's Emergency Plan for AIDS Relief, which would fund ARV treatment for millions of HIV-positive people in Africa. He asked Congress to appropriate $15 billion over the next five years. "This nation can lead the world in sparing innocent people from a plague of nature," Bush (2003) said. The program came to be known as PEPFAR, and its impact on the epidemic, and on AMPATH, would be profound.

By the end of that year, Kimaiyo was the director of AMPATH, and AMPATH was Kenya's largest provider of HIV prevention and treatment services. Indiana University and Moi University physicians had jointly authored several research papers documenting their efforts, and Kimaiyo was invited to Europe to explain how AMPATH had managed to establish and sustain a treatment program even before low-cost drugs had made treatment feasible. Other programs were just ramping up, but AMPATH was providing experience-based lessons for the world. That leadership was rewarded with funding from the US government and private foundations.

AMPATH's first award from PEPFAR, in March 2004, was approximately $6.5 million. In 2007, AMPATH was awarded a $60 million grant, and the IU School of Medicine's efforts contributed another $6 million over the five years of the grant. "USAID made the grant to the AMPATH program because of its success in developing and implementing treatment and prevention programs in Kenya for the past decade," said Ms. Henrietta Fore, the administrator of USAID at the time (Indiana University 2007). The project had gone from treating a few hundred HIV-positive patients in 2003 to more than fifty-two thousand in 2007. Bob Einterz, the principal investigator on the grant, said, "Now, along with our Kenyan partners, we look forward to moving beyond this grant to pursue our groundbreaking mission of home-based counseling and testing, and expand beyond HIV to tackle maternal and infant mortality" (Indiana University 2007). At a moment when others might have reveled in the success of the moment, Bob and his partners in AMPATH were looking for ways to return to the original mission of providing community healthcare more broadly defined.

AMPATH used the funding from PEPFAR and donations from individuals and private foundations to continue their fight against the epidemic. Over the years, AMPATH has received four cycles of USAID-PEPFAR funding for HIV care. The first two were managed by IU as the fiscal administrator, but in 2013, MTRH became the first public African institution to be the prime grant recipient of this type and level of funding and in November 2021 it again received major PEPFAR/USAID grants. As the geographic footprint of AMPATH's HIV program has grown over time, nearly all of western Kenya has benefited from AMPATH's efforts.

But the healthcare challenges of the region were not limited to HIV/AIDS. By 2010, with the HIV epidemic prevalence rate stabilizing and the rates of new infections declining, AMPATH determined they had the capacity to return to their original mission of providing generalized community healthcare. By then, the project had added additional collaborators in a consortium of North American medical programs—including Brown University in Rhode Island, the University of Chicago in Illinois, Lehigh Valley Hospital in Pennsylvania, Portland-Providence Hospital in Oregon, and the University of Toronto in Ontario, Canada—that would lend additional expertise to areas of care in addition to HIV/AIDS. These universities were heavily engaged in research, and as a result, AMPATH went from having just one funded research study in 2004 to nearly one hundred by 2010. A name change was in order. The acronym stayed the same, but it now stood for the Academic Model for Providing Access to Healthcare. To this day, HIV prevention, treatment, and support remain key components of the partnership, but the scope of the mission and the list of collaborators have grown considerably. AMPATH was to be reenvisioned.

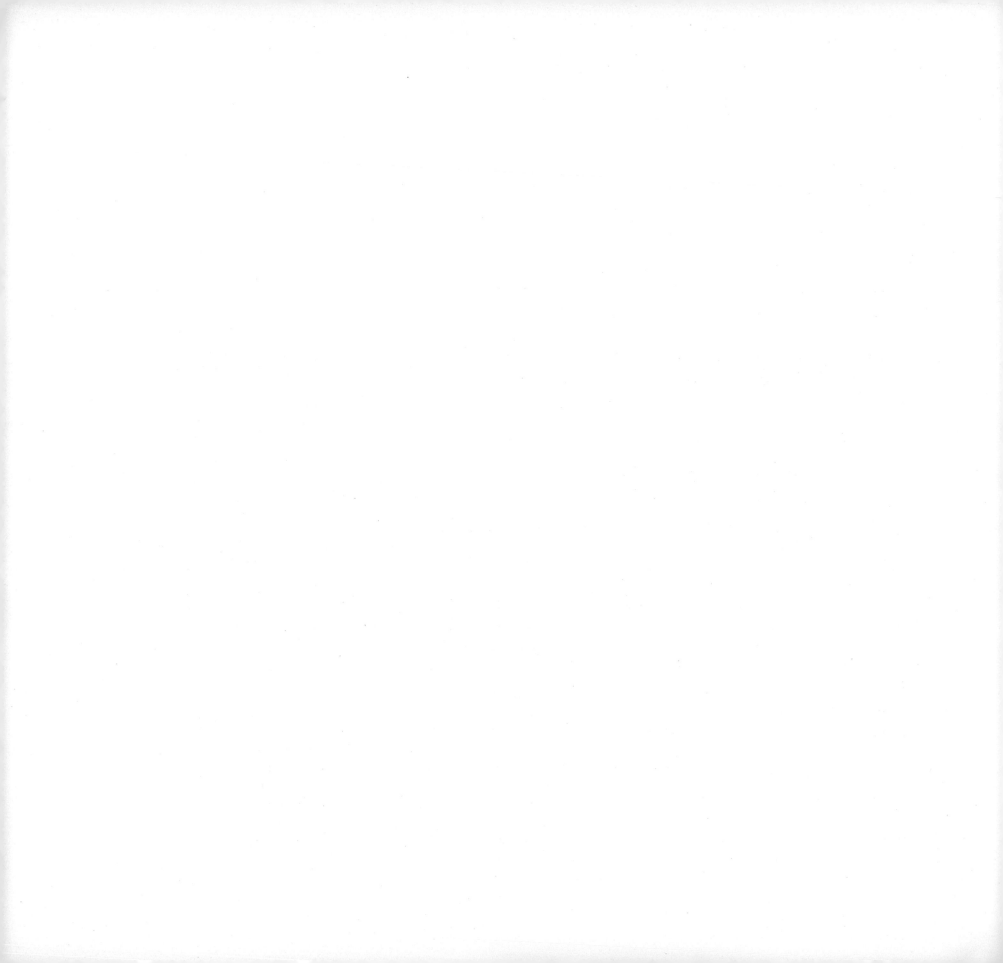

CHAPTER THREE

AMPATH Reenvisioned

Throughout the HIV/AIDS crisis, AMPATH adhered to the basic academic model based on the tripartite mission of service, education, and research, even amid the challenges of delivering healthcare in a low-income setting during an ongoing epidemic. It also continued to follow the fundamental principle that Haroun Mengech, Bob Einterz, Joe Mamlin, and the other founders first embraced: that strong healthcare systems are built on the integrity of mutually beneficial and respectful relationships at all levels. The overwhelming majority of the total staff had always been Kenyan, but leadership positions had been administered in partnership. Codirectors—one Kenyan and one Hoosier—led various projects with specific focuses. And while IU remained the primary partner of the consortium as AMPATH expanded, foreign collaborators were increasingly as likely to be from Canada, Rhode Island, Utah, or North Carolina as from the Midwest. Regardless of where people came from, individual relationships among them and people in Eldoret remained the bedrock of the operation.

In 2010, AMPATH changed its name to stand for the Academic Model Providing Access to Healthcare. After nearly a decade of building infrastructure to deliver HIV care, the leadership had identified five central themes from their collaboration over the previous decade that spoke to the need for a comprehensive, integrated, community-centered, and financially sustainable delivery model of population healthcare.

First, there was a significant chronic disease burden other than just HIV. Second, the existing health system infrastructure was fragmented, weak, and ill-equipped to manage chronic illness across the disease continuum and throughout the life course. Third, there was insufficient activity designed to promote health and prevent disease at the community level. Fourth, health sector activities were poorly responsive to the broader socioeconomic determinants of health, and limited in scope in their efforts to address poverty as a fundamental cause of health inequities. And fifth, a pathway to universal health coverage was needed as perpetual donor-funded models of care were unsustainable. (Mercer et al. 2018, 47)

During the 2010s, the reenvisioned AMPATH expanded its focus beyond HIV to noncommunicable chronic diseases and addressed population health more broadly. There was great need among patients with hypertension, diabetes, sickle cell anemia, cancer, and mental health concerns, but the MTRH staff were not sufficiently trained in these areas. AMPATH leaders were determined to not fall into the traditional disease-specific silos typical in global health and worked diligently to adhere to their model and focus on strengthening the health system as a whole and improving population health. "Population health" would become the new watch phrase. It was defined as a "responsive, equitable, and integrated system of service delivery, inclusive of health promotion, disease prevention, treatment, rehabilitation, and palliation, aimed at improving health by comprehensively addressing the biological, social, and structural determinants of health using a community-centered approach for a defined geographic population" (Mercer et al. 2018, 45–46). In somewhat less academic terms, the goal was to approach healthcare holistically and comprehensively, so all who lived within the reach of AMPATH were treated as people deserving of lifelong care and not simply subjects to be examined, studied, and treated.

Just one example of this holistic approach was the way chronic disease management was integrated into the existing home-based HIV counseling and testing program. Just being tested for HIV could carry stigma, so AMPATH had trained its staff to go into individual homes in the villages and farms around Eldoret, where privacy could be assured. Adding testing for hypertension and diabetes

to these visits ensured that neighbors were even less likely to suspect the visit had anything to do with AIDS. They instead assumed it was simply beneficial healthcare. By 2017, nearly fifteen thousand patients were being treated for hypertension and diabetes because of this new testing protocol.

As the consortium of academic institutions expanded, so did the number of private-sector and government-agency partners. Cancer had become a leading cause of premature death in sub-Saharan Africa, and the Center of Excellence in Oncology is an early example of the ways the partnership was expanding to provide clinical care, training, and research. The Moi and IU medical schools joined with Pfizer pharmaceutical, USAID, the Levinson Foundation, and three more of the consortium's university members to expand funding for care in this critical area. By 2013, the Oncology Department was housed in a new ten-bed unit at the MTRH built with the assistance of Duke University, a consortium member. About one thousand patients are now treated every month at the MTRH unit and thirteen rural clinical sites, and more than forty-five oncology doctors, nurses, and physician assistants have completed training.

Similarly, a Center for Cardiovascular and Pulmonary Disease was established in 2013 and housed in a newly constructed cardiac care unit on the MTRH campus with funding from the Hock Family Foundation and the Duke University Hubert-Yeargan Center for Global Health. The Riley Mother Baby Hospital of Kenya, also on the MTRH campus, was built in 2009 with funding from Dr. James A. Lemons, a physician at the Riley Hospital for Children at Indiana University Health in Indianapolis. Today, it provides for the delivery of twenty thousand newborn babies a year, has operating rooms for an average of sixteen cesarean deliveries every day, and has one of the largest functioning neonatal intensive care units in all of East

Africa, with an average daily census of about one hundred critically ill newborn infants. Both facilities were named after the Indiana children's poet James Whitcomb Riley.

Many other initiatives were started or expanded during the third decade of the partnership, but two that perhaps speak most clearly of the holistic approach taken over the entire history of AMPATH are those focused on agriculture and technology. Neither is immediately associated with healthcare, but both figure prominently in the organization's approach to treating the whole person.

Early in the HIV/AIDS epidemic, doctors realized the ARV drugs they were prescribing were not always producing the dramatic "Lazarus effects" they anticipated. Malnutrition was the reason, so AMPATH clinicians started to prescribe food along with the ARVs. That food was eventually produced by six farms supported in part by donations from the Howard G. Buffett Foundation. HIV-positive clients of AMPATH worked the agricultural fields to produce tons of fresh produce that was supplemented with cooking oil and grains donated by the World Food Program. As patients collected their weekly rations, the effectiveness of the ARVs was greatly enhanced. In addition, some clients already on ARVs were hired to work at the farms and the distribution warehouse.

Today, the AMPATH farms are all closed, and food distribution, like the World Food Program, has ended. Clients were becoming dependent on the handouts, and there were concerns that people would intentionally contract HIV to gain access to the food. The AMPATH Safety Net program shifted its focus to helping people grow their own food and providing training on financial planning and farming practices. As a result, clients were able to save money and buy the agricultural inputs needed to increase yields on their small plots and gardens. AMPATH currently partners with several international organizations to enhance these efforts, including a partnership with

Corteva Agriscience, the agricultural division of Dow-DuPont. Corteva donates employee time and other resources to maintain two dozen demonstration plots in the area that help farmers learn how to improve their cropping and business techniques on farms as small as a single acre. The Safety Net works with more than eighty different farmer groups across western Kenya.

Since AMPATH's inception, health information technology (HIT) has been a key innovation in support of the overall healthcare mission. As soon as AMPATH began seeing patients, computerized systems were developed to maintain client records. Initially, healthcare workers carried personal digital assistants (PDAs) into the field, assigning each client a unique number that followed them even as they shifted from one household to another. The data in those very small handheld computers was uploaded each night into a mainframe on the IUPUI campus. In 2013, the PDAs were replaced by mobile phones and the data-storage computers were relocated to the MTRH campus. Today, the AMPATH Medical Record System (AMRS) is supported by IU's Regenstrief Institute and is deployed at the AMPATH center in Eldoret and forty other clinical sites in East Africa. The AMRS is one of the first and largest examples of an electronic medical record system in sub-Saharan Africa. To date, the AMRS has collected more than two hundred million discrete clinical observations from 3.5 million AMPATH visits made by eight hundred thousand enrolled patients. Stored data includes confidential information such as test results; patient descriptors such as symptoms, vital signs, and physical exam findings; and diagnoses and treatments from clinical encounters.

Efforts like these and many others distinguish AMPATH as a model for collaborative development efforts between universities in the developed and developing world. To better understand themselves and consolidate their vision across the now much larger organization, in 2018 AMPATH conducted an exhaustive analysis that described how it had leveraged the power of partnerships to build the holistic, community care–centered collaboration it had become. The comprehensive population health model now includes clinical programs covering adult and pediatric HIV; prevention of mother-to-child transmission of HIV; maternal, neonatal, and child health; family planning; tuberculosis; diabetes; hypertension; cardiovascular disease; anticoagulation; oncology; palliative care; mental health; and several crosscutting departments, including human resources and administration; grants management; pharmacy; laboratory; informatics; food and income security; monitoring and evaluation; quality improvement; and research (Mercer et al. 2018, 49).

Using a unique methodology, leadership from the MoH, the MTRH, the MUCHS, AMPATH, and other stakeholders created an infographic and conceptual illustration called a "learning map" that represented the AMPATH vision and strategy (see image in chap. 5). The map was used to spread the vison of population health throughout the catchment area of one million people in western Kenya. Over several months, nearly one thousand AMPATH and MoH staff from all different roles in the system met to discuss and understand the map and the ideas it represented. It was also presented to approximately thirty high-level executives from various pharmaceutical companies and foundations, the Gates Foundation, the National Institutes of Health, and USAID-PEPFAR to share the vision with these key partners and funders. Continuing efforts are aimed at setting measurable goals and objectives along with implementation schedules.

Maintaining awareness of this vision and strategy across such a wide-ranging and comprehensive program is no small challenge, but it is hardly the first challenge faced by AMPATH. Fundamentally, it is an effort to consolidate, sustain, and encourage the esprit de corps that has motivated the AMPATH staff since that very first meeting in 1988.

A Calling to Serve

Since the independence movements of the 1960s, sub-Saharan Africa—like most of the developing world—has devoted considerable resources to the education of healthcare workers only to see sizable numbers of them migrate to the developed world, taking their knowledge and skills with them. Roughly half of sub-Saharan African countries suffer an annual loss of more than 30 percent of the doctors they train. This equates to tens of thousands of doctors. Roughly equal numbers of nurses from the region also emigrate to developed countries (Kasper and Bajunirwe 2012). Kenya fares somewhat better than its African neighbors, but recent estimates are that 30 to 40 percent of the country's six hundred medical graduates each year leave after completing their internship (Muraguri 2015) and that one in every five nurses trained in Kenya applies to emigrate (Otieno 2016).

The core motivations for emigration of health workers are financial incentives, career development opportunities, and problematic management according to Willis-Shattuck and colleagues, who found that "recognition is highly influential in health worker motivation and that adequate resources and appropriate infrastructure can improve morale significantly" (2008, 247). When positive reinforcement in the form of institutional support is absent, the combined effects of low and inconsistent pay, long working hours, and poor working conditions can lead to burnout syndrome. Angela Oketch (2019) of the *Daily Nation* newspaper recently reported about the experience of a medical school graduate who enthusiastically took on an assignment in rural Kenya only to quickly become overwhelmed by lack of equipment, inadequate staffing, and a feeling of isolation from peers. "I was never prepared for such reality. I had no idea what I was going to meet in the wards," he said. His desire to serve his country where his skills were most needed was thwarted by material conditions that left him feeling alone and unsupported.

And yet, there is but "scanty information about the syndrome among medical workers in Kenya," according to a study headed by Kokonya (2014, 14) conducted at the Kenyatta National Hospital (KNH) in Nairobi. The study is one of only a few to look directly at burnout as a reason medical doctors leave the country. The authors noted that studies on burnout syndrome among medical workers in Europe and the United States have demonstrated that all cadres of health personnel suffer from various levels of burnout syndrome. Their analysis of doctors, nurses, technicians, and others in healthcare at Kenya's premier medical center found the rate of burnout syndrome was 95.4 percent—a shockingly high percentage even when compared to British Columbia (55%), Austria (58%), and North England (66%). The major contributor to burnout intensity scores at KNH was work environment (56%).

While burnout is not the only factor contributing to emigration of medical personnel, it is surely a major factor. Research suggests that improvements in the quality of facilities, increases in staffing, and greater institutional support are most often identified as key to decreasing burnout and increasing job satisfaction. Interestingly, Kasprowicz and colleagues (2020) argue that strengthening African-led health research capacity in sub-Saharan Africa is the most optimal approach to increasing retention of medical experts, arguing that these collaborations with colleagues contribute to enhanced self-worth as well as improved working conditions and patient outcomes. It may be that these research opportunities partially mitigate

the enthusiasm for emigration to satisfy career objectives (Poppe et al. 2014).

Kenya has made progress in staunching the outflow of its trained medical providers. For example, 939 nurses were verified to apply for foreign registration in 2003, but just 262 did so in 2013, according to a Nursing Council of Kenya (NCK) database from 2014 (as referenced in Brownie and Oywer 2016). The prospect for improving the material conditions of Kenyan healthcare facilities has been enhanced by the devolution of national revenue control. In 2010, the newly ratified constitution created forty-seven semi-autonomous county governments, and in 2013, healthcare and other services were transferred from the central government to these counties. This transition sought to strengthen democracy and accountability, increase community participation, improve efficiency, and reduce inequities. Early indications are that while an initial lack of clarity over the specific roles and responsibilities of county and national governments was partially responsible for healthcare worker strikes and other disruptions, by 2017, counties were exercising increased decision-making and allocating new funding to facilities and capacity improvements (Tsofa et al. 2017).

AMPATH's ability to retain its highly qualified staff predates devolution and the new constitution, however. The leadership has been able to employ innovative methods to retain its doctors and nurses in large measure because of its collaborative relationship with the Ministry of Health's Moi Teaching and Referral Hospital. Staff have regularly held joint appointments between the two that facilitate enhanced pay schemes and more engaging duties, often working side by side with North Americans in the consortium.

A 2007 study led by Tom Inui of the Regenstrief Institute at the IU School of Medicine in Indianapolis provided clear evidence of the benefits of AMPATH's collaborative environment. They found that staff were motivated first and foremost by a desire to serve their patients and clients and that staff recognized that this was possible because they worked in an organization that made it easy for them to connect with colleagues, to avoid crises, and to consistently make a positive difference in the lives of their fellow community members. They commented on the importance of their work being recognized by leaders in the organization and even by colleagues outside Kenya. They said AMPATH allowed them to grow as individuals and professionals without having to leave their home country, all while directly contributing to a mission that served their nation.

Tom Inui and colleagues (2007) observe that "the philosophic foundations of the program are easily identified in the interviews. Program personnel, from top to bottom, feel 'called' by a service ideology. They particularly recognize the need to respond to the most vulnerable populations, including the sickest and poorest individuals in western Kenya: children, orphans, widows, and others. There is an explicit, shared belief in the need to put these individuals and their care first" (Inui et al. 2007, 1748). More recent theoretical discussion among organizational researchers provides additional ways to think about these motivations, and much attention has centered on notions of calling as a service ideology.

Organizational psychologists have developed a substantial literature devoted to the study of work and generally conclude that work constitutes a sizable part of the subjective quality of life (Loscocco and Roschelle 1991). Wrzesniewski and colleagues (1997) identified three attitudes toward work: as a job (focus on financial rewards and necessity rather than pleasure or fulfillment; not a major positive part of life), as a career (focus on advancement), or as a calling (focus on enjoyment of fulfilling, socially useful work). While not mutually exclusive and clearly related to job satisfaction, pay, supervision, benefits, promotional structure, and coworkers, they found that respondents who saw their work as a calling had the highest life and work satisfaction. More recent studies into the calling distinction by Duffy and Dik (2013) found that the links among career commitment, work meaning, job satisfaction, life meaning, and life satisfaction were most robust when individuals were actually living out their calling at work. Duffy and colleagues (2017) also found that individuals with greater access to vocational opportunity and income security showed the highest levels of the calling motivation and life satisfaction.

Throughout my time in Eldoret, I was listening for confirmation of the insights Tom Inui and his colleagues discovered about the motivations of the AMPATH staff more than a decade earlier. Would the service ideology they identified persist in an era where HIV is a chronic condition treated effectively across all segments of society instead of a raging health emergency demanding urgent attention? Would AMPATH workers still say their jobs were satisfying because they were making a positive difference for the community? Did they still feel recognized by their leaders as people who were not just working but responding to a calling that motivated them to greater achievement? And if so, was this true of just a small handful of people fortunate enough to come in regular close contact with foreign experts, or was it true among workers who rarely saw a North American or even the preeminent confines of high-level medical facilities and university classrooms in Eldoret? AMPATH workers were kind enough to let me know, over and over again, as the following chapters attest.

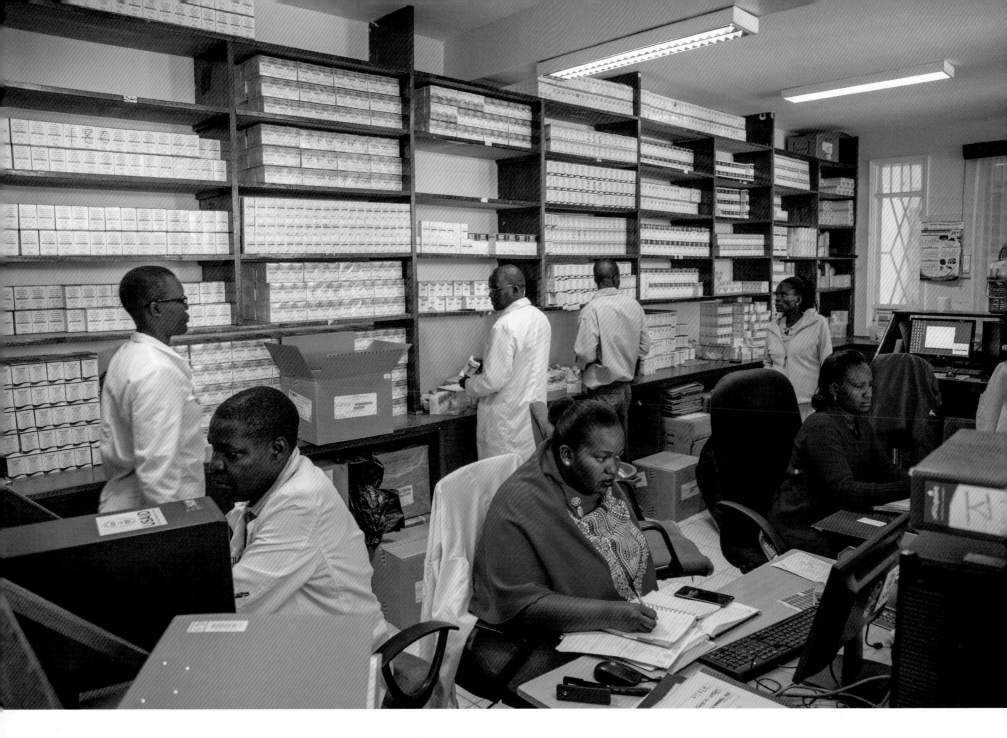

Pharmacists and assistants
work in the main pharmacy
on the ground floor of
the AMPATH Centre on
Nandi Road in Eldoret.

PART TWO

PHOTOGRAPHIC ESSAYS
OF WORKERS

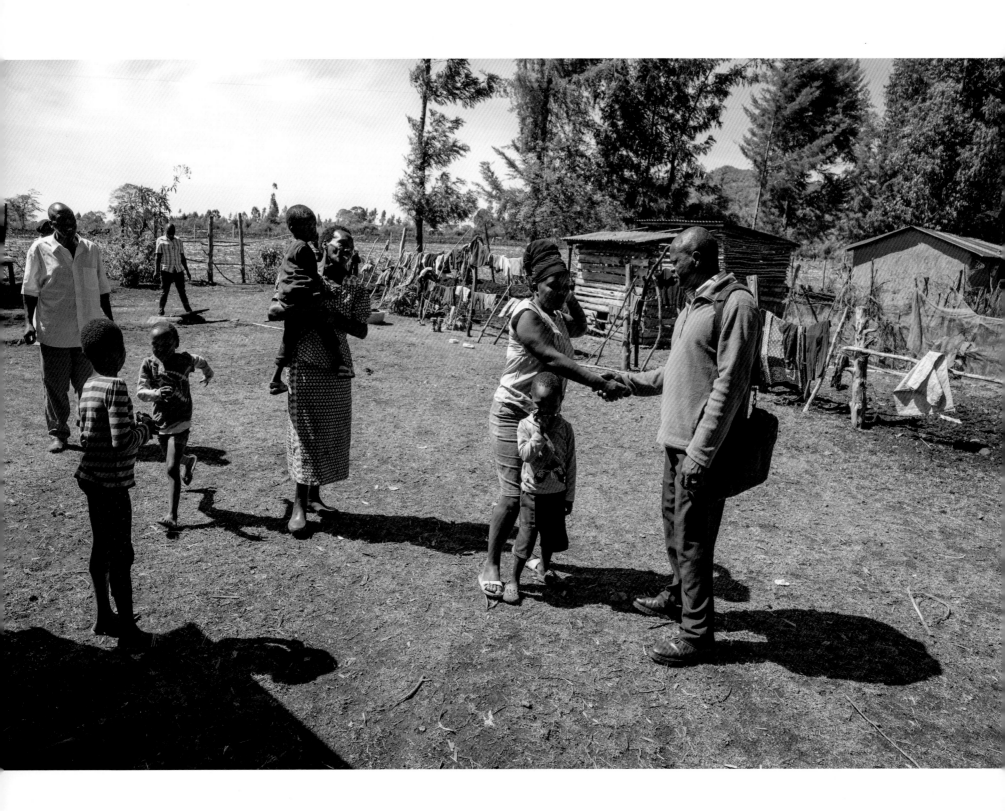

CHAPTER FOUR

Population Health through Economic Empowerment

Anyara Papa Helps People Help Themselves in Turbo

Mr. Givinal Papa Anyara remembers the day he began working for AMPATH quite well—Sunday, February 12, 2006. The HIV epidemic was filling the wards of the district hospital in Busia County, just as it was filling wards across East Africa. By then, 2.2 million Africans had died from the disease, and more than 3 million were newly infected that year. AIDS was the leading cause of death in sub-Saharan Africa, and because it disproportionately affected young adults, there were thousands of orphans living with grandparents across the countryside.

Papa was not hired to diagnose illness or treat infection. He was not a doctor or nurse who could give the drugs to save their lives. His job was to help people help themselves. He taught them how to organize, pool their resources effectively, and assist each other with small loans. He taught them how to grow African leafy vegetables and other crops that could sustain them through those troubling times.

"I was hired as a business development officer to train groups on business and agriculture in Teso. I would teach groups of six members about business. All were HIV-positive people," Papa recalled. Teso is an area straddling the border between Kenya and Uganda about ninety miles west of Eldoret. "We were giving loans of 5,000 shillings to a person. [US$68 in 2006] The person was to pay it back to the group within one month, then give the money to next person. It was supposed to be a revolving fund."

Facing, Anyara Papa greets Valentine Chepkorich, the daughter of Phillip (in white shirt) and Pauline Tallam (with child in arms), who live on a small plot north of Turbo. She has used GISHE to pay school fees for her four youngest (of eight) children, three of whom have completed college. Her husband's family owns the posho mill near the road, but he is not a member of the GISHE. Papa says of men, "The problem is they don't join."

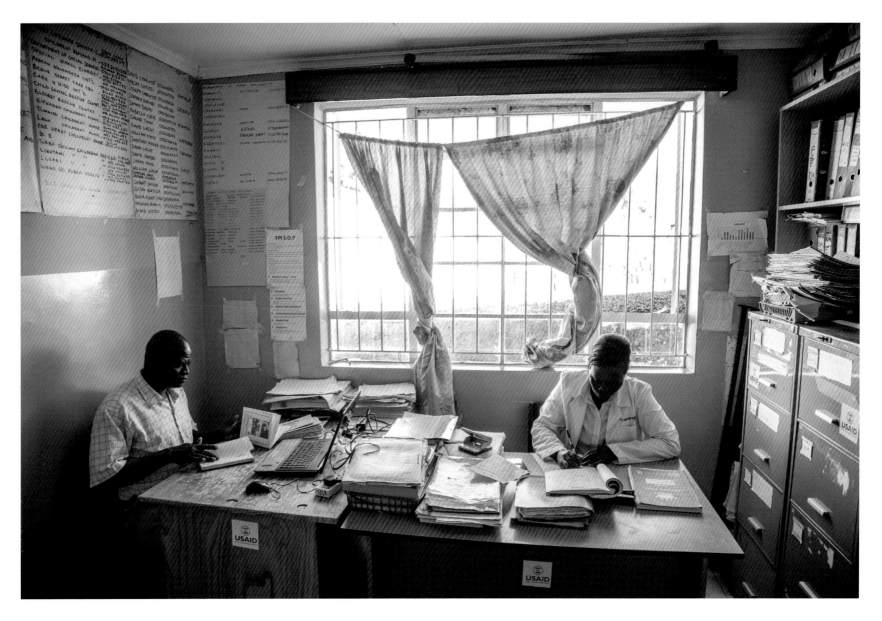

Above, Papa shares an office with Caroline Kibiego (right) and Margaret Alegwa in the AMPATH Centre, which is part of the subcounty hospital. The three collaborate daily to support nearly ten thousand people around Turbo in the counties of Uasin Gishu and Kakamega.

Facing, Schoolchildren from the Turbo Township Primary School play near the subcounty hospital in Turbo.

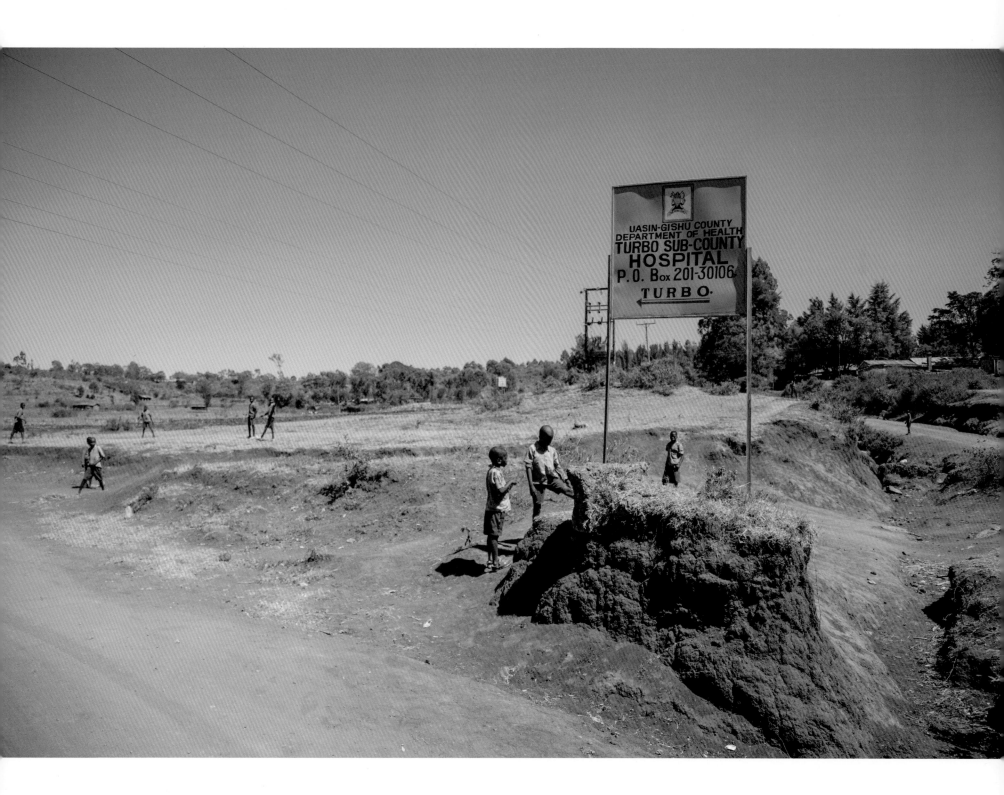

Anyara Papa at his desk in
the AMPATH clinic in Turbo.

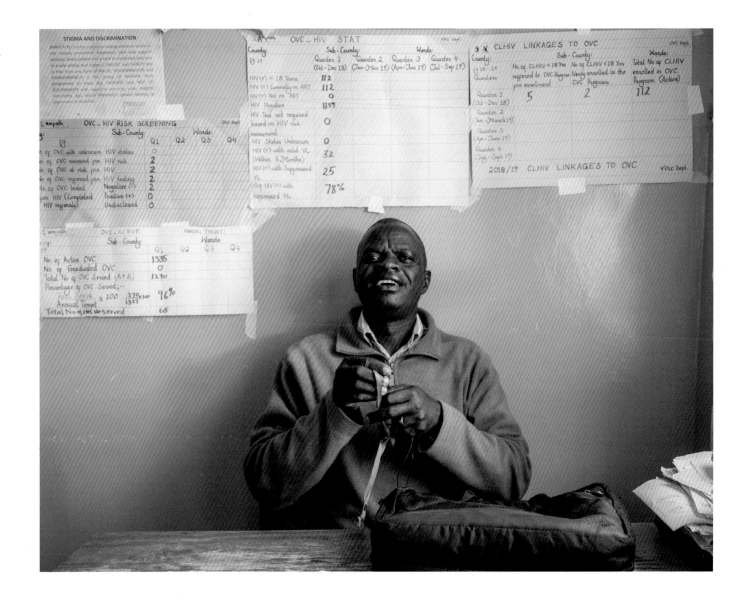

"Unfortunately, the program did not pick up well," he confided. Like so many AMPATH-sponsored projects, success was not immediate. The idea was to inject money into capital-starved areas and increase savings rates. But Papa and his Family Preservation Initiative (FPI) colleagues soon realized people had little reason to pay back the loan. There was no pressure on the borrower from the others in the group because no one else had a claim to the money. It wasn't theirs, so it didn't matter that it didn't come back to the group. "So, we started the GISHE program in 2009, and I started training both business and agriculture skills." Money without attendant social responsibility to the community did not solve the problem. GISHE did.

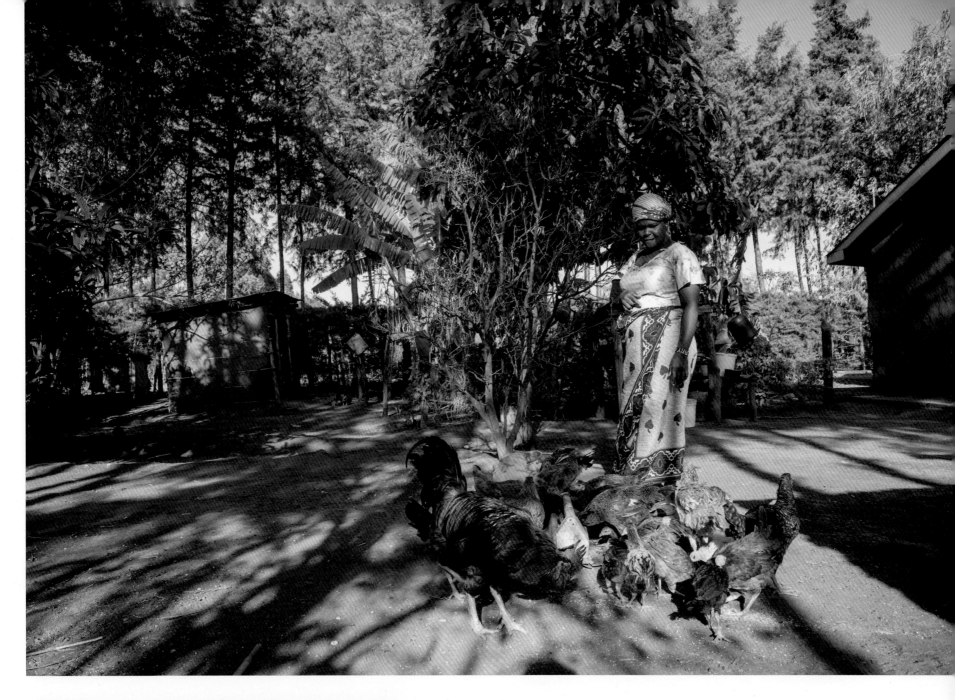

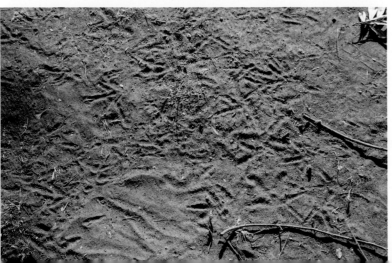

Above and left, Elizabeth Nanyama has been a GISHE member for about six years. She participated in a poultry project AMPATH conducted in collaboration with Dow Agriculture (Corteva) and now sells eggs at a roadside stand in front of her house. She started with nine chicks and ended up with sixty-nine laying hens.

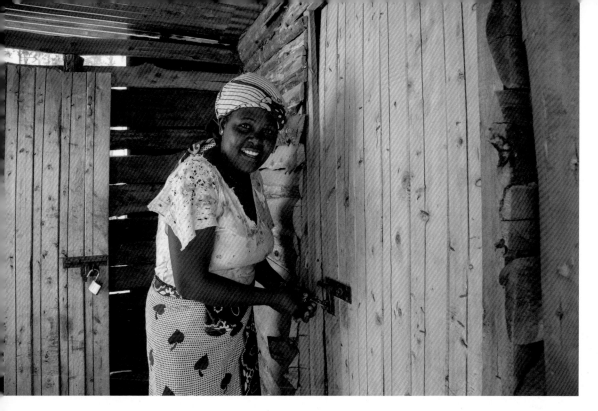

GISHE

GISHE stands for Group Integrated Savings for Health and Empowerment. Like the groups Papa had started earlier, all members of a group lived close to each other in the same village. All were HIV-positive clients of AMPATH, and most were women widowed by AIDS. "Those people we gave the money to in the initial stage, they did not do it well. But there was one lady who also cooperated with a social worker, and that worked very well. We gave her some money, and she started selling bananas and assorted fruits," he recalled. "After selling them for a while, she changed the business and started buying cassava from the farms and taking them to markets in nearby towns. She was able to buy a plot of her own and built a permanent house." Her success required coordination between Papa and the social worker. The key seemed to be the acquisition of business knowledge while working within a social support network.

GISHE turned out to be the solution AMPATH needed. Papa has been training groups about business, proposal writing, accounting, interest, project evaluation, and other business practices, but he has also helped them build the social network required to sustain economic activity. The GISHE groups work like a community bank and are called "table banks." Members contribute to the bank and keep meticulous records of who has how much in and who has how much out. Interest rates are less than half what an actual bank would charge, and the loan amounts are much smaller than what actual banks are willing to offer. Borrowers repay the loans because the money belongs to the people who live next door or down the road. There is social obligation to repay but also a social incentive to succeed in whatever venture the money underwrites.

"At the same time we were forming the GISHE groups, the social workers were setting up social groups" based on

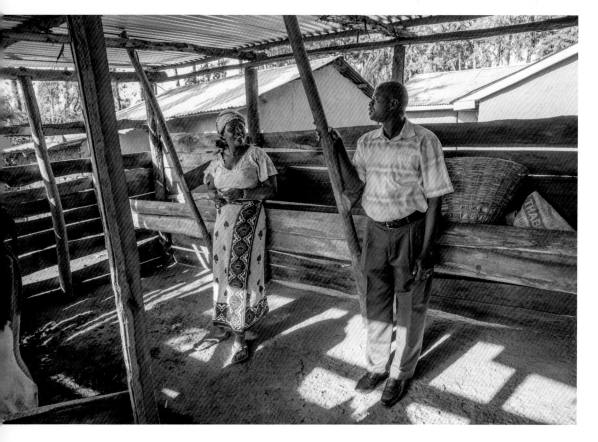

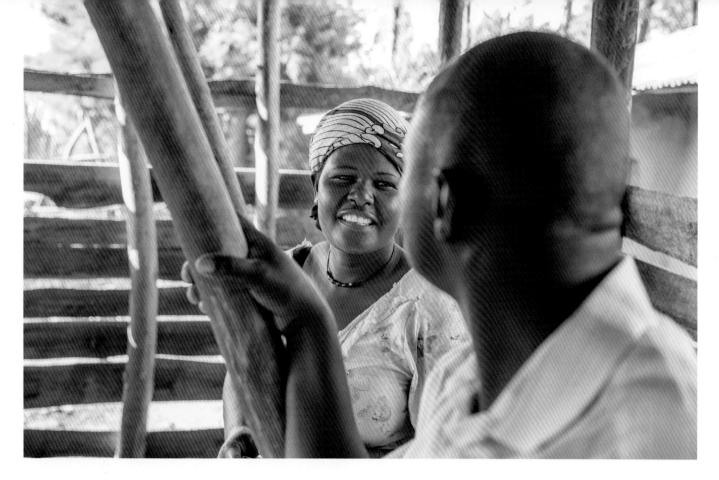

Facing and left, To start her small farm, Elizabeth initially bought a goat using GISHE money, then sold it to get a calf, and now she has two cows and a newborn calf. She bought enough grass and grain to feed them during the dry season and therefore has no need for grazing, which requires much more land than she has on her small plot. All along the way, Elizabeth consulted with Papa. She says, "My GISHE has been very good for my family and me."

their knowledge of the community, he said. "The social worker would refer the groups to me, and I would train them on GISHE and table banking and business skills." He continued, "It worked better because the clients were coming to the clinic. After being screened by the nurse, and then seeing the doctor, they would be sent back to the social worker, who would stabilize them and get them in a group. We were sharing our office with the OVC [the initiative to assist orphans and vulnerable children] social worker, and we could work together."

Papa was still sharing an office with two social workers, Ms. Margaret Alegwa and Ms. Caroline Kibiego, when I met with him in 2019 at the AMPATH clinic in Turbo. Together, they worked with more than three hundred GISHE groups around Turbo in Usain Gishu and Kakamega counties, but Papa no longer trained the group members himself. Instead, he trained and supervised

thirty group empowerment service providers (GESPs), who, in turn, trained new groups as the program expanded to encourage enrollment in the National Hospital Insurance Fund—Kenya's mechanism for building a national healthcare system. Papa has seen a lot of adaptation and change over his years with AMPATH.

Homeland of the Iteso People

For Papa, it all began in his home area of Teso, the traditional homeland of the Iteso people, who currently live on both sides of the Kenya-Uganda border. The town of Busia, also straddling the border, is the main city. Busia is just eighty miles from Eldoret, but fifteen years ago, it was a long three-hour drive. AMPATH's efforts out there on the border were a pretty big stretch for an organization that had, until then, worked within an hour or so from the MTRH. Papa's boss at the time was Mr. Benjamin Andama, head of the FPI, which was one of a half dozen projects AMPATH created to support people living with HIV. This idea that healthcare ought to include community support has animated the collaboration since the first meeting between Haroun Mengech and the visitors from Indiana in 1998. By the time the HIV crisis was hitting full stride, it was perhaps only logical that those old ideas were still part of the solution.

Papa has turned those ideas into action, and he has done so for a generation now. The distinctive feature of AMPATH is that it has always been about more than HIV testing and treatment. Early on, they realized that positive people also needed maternal and child health and nutrition counseling, as well as finance assistance, if they were to survive the virus. Papa's job is helping patients gain financial stability and independence so they can manage their healthcare, whether they are HIV positive or negative.

AMPATH's initial goal was to confront the AIDS epidemic, and Papa joined the fight when program efforts were new and untested. Like Joe Mamlin, Sylvester Kimaiyo, Bob Einterz, and other medical leaders, he has seen the organization transform from a tight focus on the HIV epidemic to a broader focus on chronic healthcare and now to the even grander goal of universal healthcare. Unlike those doctors, however, Papa has no medical credentials and no university degree. He spends almost no time at the grand tertiary care hospital in Eldoret. His days are spent on a motorcycle plying the red-dirt roads around Turbo, meeting with GESPs and GISHE groups in tin-roofed churches or visiting clients in their small houses, where they grow African vegetables and raise chickens on quarter-acre plots located a long walk from the road. This was true when he was in Busia, and has

remained true since he moved to Turbo in 2012—he has always worked with rural people, and they know him well.

Because he has been with AMPATH for so long, Papa knows what the transition from AMPATH treating AIDS to AMPATH pursuing population health really means for the common person. Organizational structures put in place to address the AIDS crisis worked very well, and the lessons learned have paid dividends that are being applied to address the even larger goals of universal healthcare financed by a national health insurance plan.

A Widow Back Home in Lumakanda

Ms. Ebby Opisa is a widow. As a young woman of eighteen in 1995, she married a Luo man, left her Luhya family in the village of Lumakanda just west of Turbo near the Lugari Forest, and moved down near Lake Victoria. She was sixty miles from home, living with people of a different tribe and learning how to be a good wife. In 1998, her husband died of AIDS, and Ebby tested positive for HIV shortly after. She had no children, so returned to her family home only to see her brother die of AIDS two years later. Left her alone on her parents' small plot of land, she struggled to feed herself. By 2003, her CD4 count was less than two hundred—the threshold for a diagnosis of AIDS. Ebby worried that she too would die.

When she had tested positive five years earlier, there was not much else to do. There was no cure. There were no medicines to take. She had a place to live, but over time the virus in her body multiplied, killing the white blood cells that protected her from infection and making her weak. Ebby eventually became so sick that she walked five miles to the subcounty hospital in Turbo and was immediately sent to the newly constructed AMPATH clinic just next door. They prescribed her the antiretroviral drugs

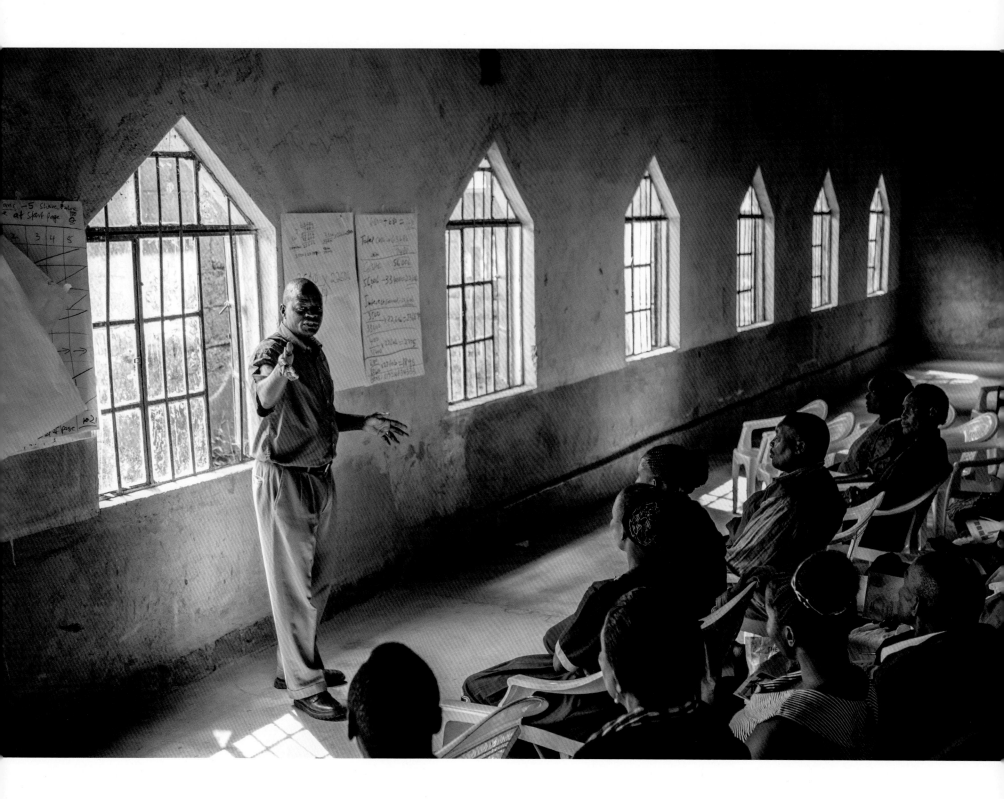

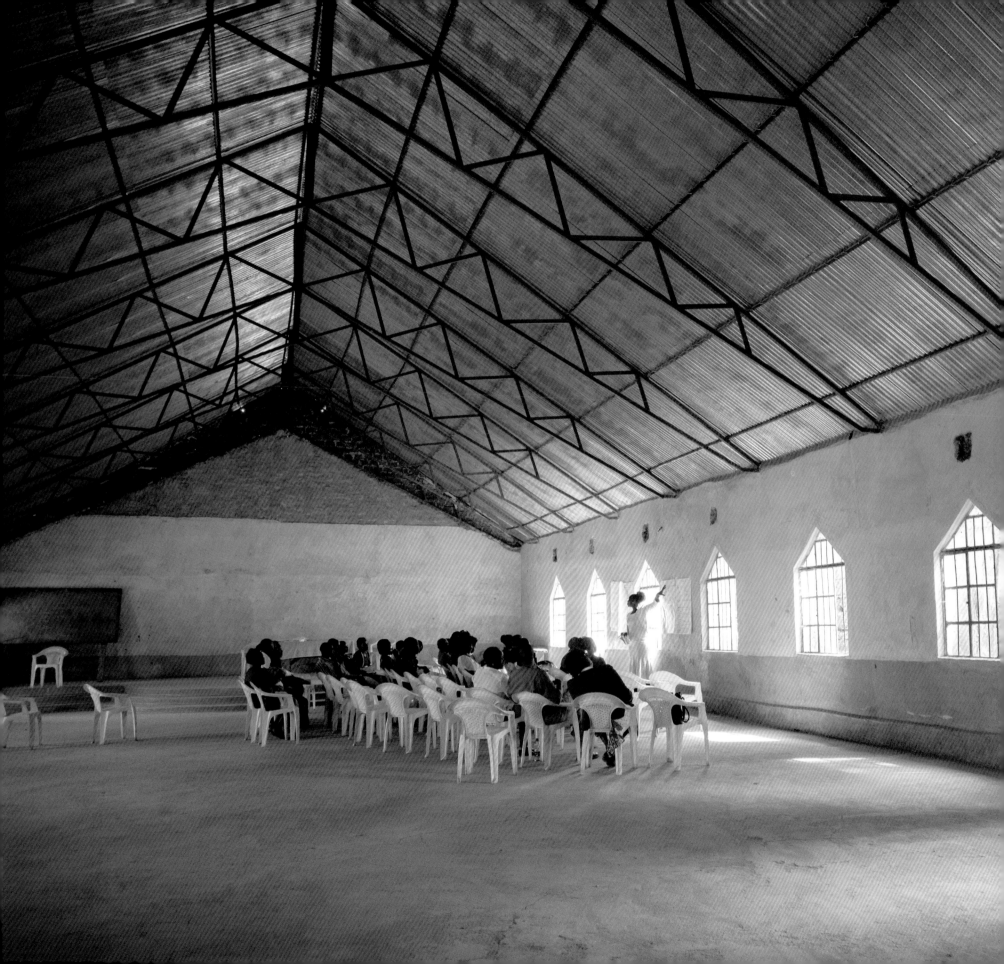

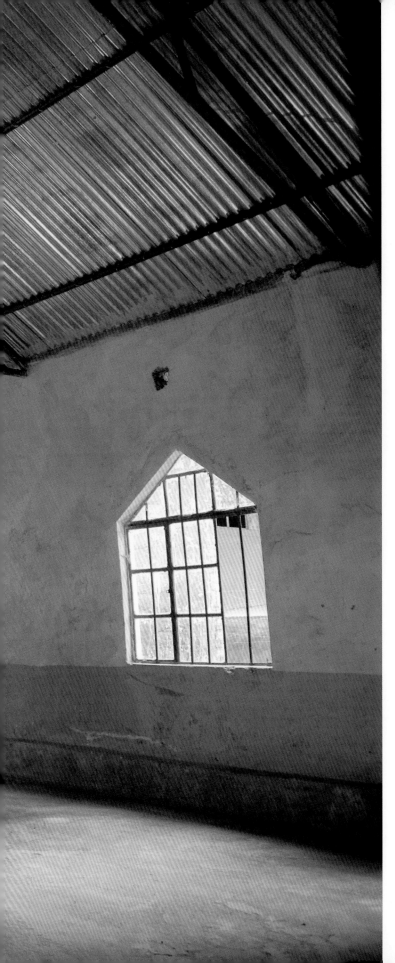

that interrupted the virus's reproduction and allowed her body to regain its strength.

But recovery required more than just drugs. She was sent to the social worker, and then she was sent to Papa. Papa recognize the entrepreneurial spirit in Ebby and worked with her and her neighbors to organize the Tumaini support group—a GISHE that was then entirely composed of HIV-positive people and almost entirely female. That was 2014. Since then, Ebby has raised two children from her village who were orphaned by AIDS. She used the loans she drew from the GISHE to buy goats and eventually a cow. She sold used clothing at the market. She raised chickens, selling the eggs in the village and then the hens when they stopped laying.

Recently, she participated in a poultry project AMPATH collaborated on with Dow Agriculture (now Corteva Agriscience). The program provided two-month-old chicks to group members who would raise them to be laying hens. But because Ebby had been working with Papa for so long, she had sufficient expertise to raise "peeps" in a brooding box in her living room. Once she had them vaccinated and healthy, she supplied the chicks to others in the groups, who would then use them to start their own businesses.

"My dream is for this orphan I am taking care of. I'll make sure I sell eggs and hens to make him get his degree," she told me. "He'll go to Eldoret University. He'll pay part of his school fees and I'll pay part to achieve his dream." She recalled, "I started with him when he was in

Judith Nandwa Lubanga, a community health volunteer in Kiplombe, leads a workshop session about record keeping in the sanctuary of St. Columban's Church across the road from the AMPATH Centre. Support from longtime partner AbbVie Foundation has fueled the growth of the program since its start in 2012. Today, 84 percent of Chama cha MamaToto participants deliver their baby in a health facility, compared to 50 percent for mothers not in the program.

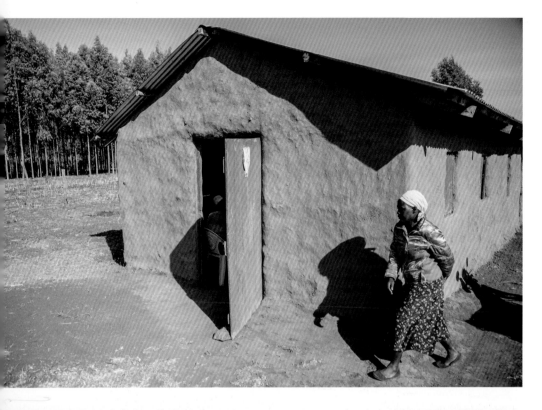

Top, A local woman arrives just before the start of the weekly meeting of the Siyenga Community Group. Her GISHE meets in a Salvation Army church about three and a half miles north of Turbo. At the time, there were thirty-one people in group: nine men and twenty-two women. Siyenga is one of the oldest groups in the area. Most of the members were either clients of AMPATH Plus or the chronic disease management program.

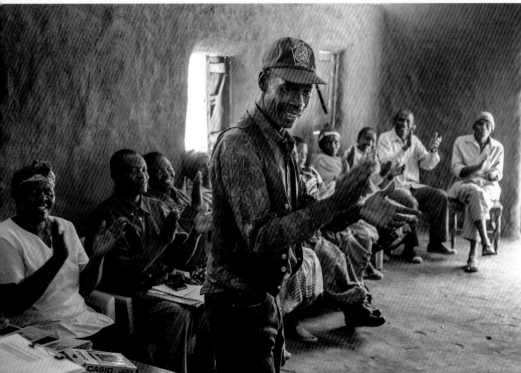

Bottom, Richard Kubani, the group's primary contact with AMPATH, is one of about thirty GESPs working for Papa to help train new groups and assist with established groups. Every GISHE elects a president, a secretary, a treasurer, and three "money handlers" to one-year terms. Most of the money placed into the group's account at the start of the meeting is distributed as loans to members by the end of each meeting. Any balance is kept in a lockbox that requires all three officers' keys to open.

class four. The parents died of HIV, and he had no one to take care of him. I said, 'I've not given back' for the care I had received from AMPATH. Let me take care of these children and I'll get blessings from God through them.'" She continued, "They lived with me when they were not in school, but right now they are in college" (a post–high school training similar to American community college). "They are doing well."

Ebby is currently a GESP. She oversees five groups and is a peer social mentor to two additional groups. On Papa's advice, Ebby saves 20 shillings (KSh) per day to pay for her monthly National Hospital Insurance Fund (NHIF) fee of KSh 500 (US$5). "Because I had the card, I could go to Lumakanda to see the doctor," she said. She recently had an operation to remove a fibroid cyst, and the cost was completely covered by NHIF. "I tell my groups to save for NHIF. It is a very good thing."

Spilling Over a Bit

Benjamin Andama was one of the first AMPATH staffers I met. In 2009, he was heading FPI and had an office in the

From AIDS to Population Health

basement of the AMPATH Centre in Eldoret. I told him of my plans to bring students to Kenya and he said "karibuni sana," meaning "you are all very welcome." He told me there were many good stories about his staff and their efforts to economically empower their clients. Two years later he put two of my students in contact with Mr. Richard Kubani and helped IU student Claire Shirley and Moi student Renaud Ocholla report a story about how GISHE provided HIV-positive people with the capital they needed to sustain their small-plot agriculture.

Many Kenyans in the Great Rift Valley are fortunate to have their own land. While some huge farms still operate as they did under white rule during colonial times, independence in 1963 gave many rural Kenyans the opportunity to claim small plots, often only a quarter acre, where they could scratch out a subsistence living. The problem today is that farmers have no clear land ownership rights and so cannot pledge the property as collateral for financing to buy the inputs needed for larger yields. Early on, however, AMPATH recognized the potential for these small farmers, and FPI has often collaborated with other initiatives focused on orphan care and food security to encourage self-sufficiency based on small-plot development.

Top, Damary Owieno, the group's president, watches over a younger member as she prepares to distribute the record books. Every member keeps a record of all transactions. On average, each member contributes about 500 shillings a week, or US$5.

Middle and bottom, The group's three "money handlers" are the only members who put their hands on the cash that is placed into the collective's account. They record every transaction in books kept with the president.

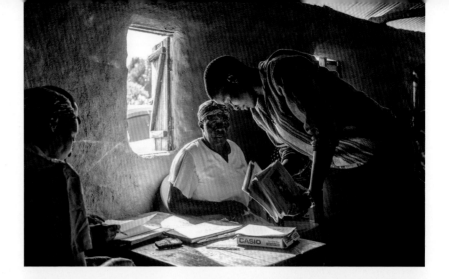
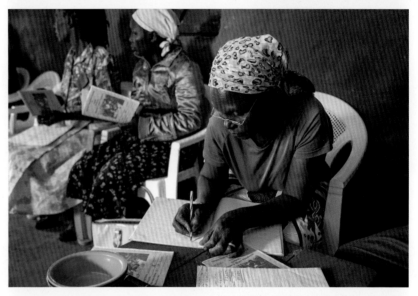
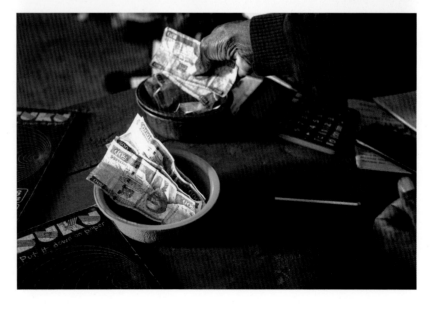

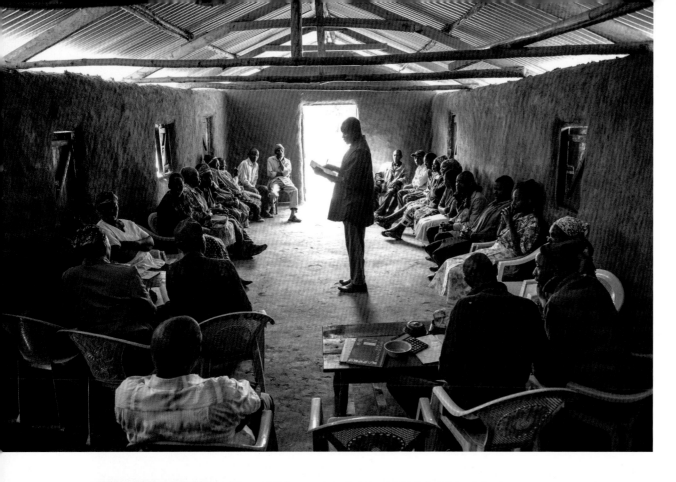

The treasurer describes the day's transactions to the group after all transactions have been completed. Each of the group's officers serve for just one year, though they can be reelected after sitting out a year.

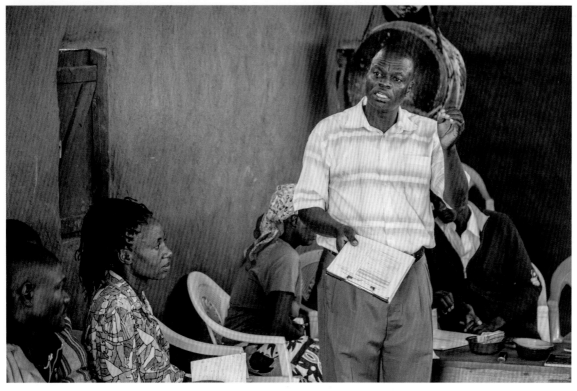

Papa talks with folks at the end of the meeting. He does not ordinarily visit a group as well organized and long established as the one in Siyenga.

At the beginning of my visits, AMPATH's organizational structures seemed straightforward. FPI was economic empowerment. OVC was orphans and vulnerable children. HHI (HAART and Harvest Initiative) supplied prescribed food. HTC was home testing and counseling. LACE (the Legal Aid Centre of Eldoret) was legal assistance. The emphasis was holistic—focused on the treatment of HIV-positive people's health in the clinical setting but also in the community. Benjamin's FPI trained people like Papa to provide the knowledge and skills their clients needed to build capital and grow their farms. By preserving the family, they preserved their patients. It appeared simple to me, but their three-letter initiative worked with the other three-letter initiatives in ways that were far more integrated and complex than I had imagined.

Ten years later, AMPATH's structure is transitioning to support the national goal of universal healthcare. Benjamin went from working for FPI to Safety Net to Population Health. The realignment is important for administrative purposes and demonstrates to funding agencies that AMPATH is prepared to work with the Ministry of Health on the expansion of NHIF. But the work is still collaborative, and the goal is still empowerment.

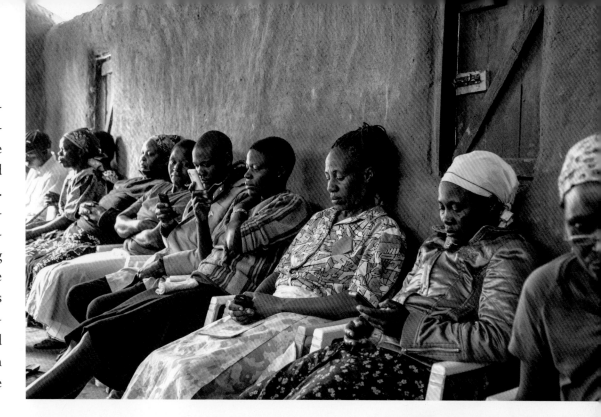

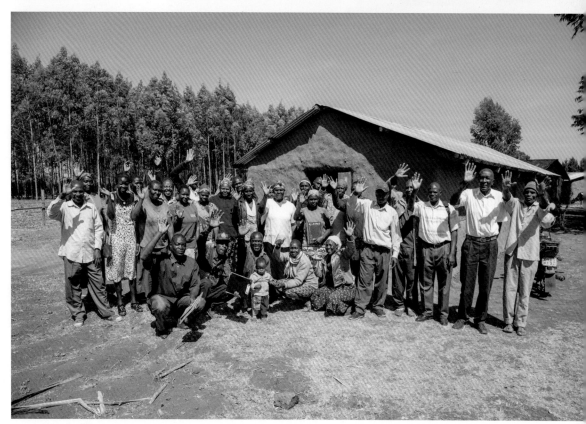

Top, Every member of the GISHE calculates transactions using their mobile phones to ensure that all agree on the amounts being contributed, allocated as loans, and repaid with interest. The interest rate GISHE charges themselves is as little as a quarter the rate a bank would charge, if a bank were willing to make such small loans.

Right, The people in Siyenga are proud of their GISHE group and community and asked me if I would make their photo before leaving.

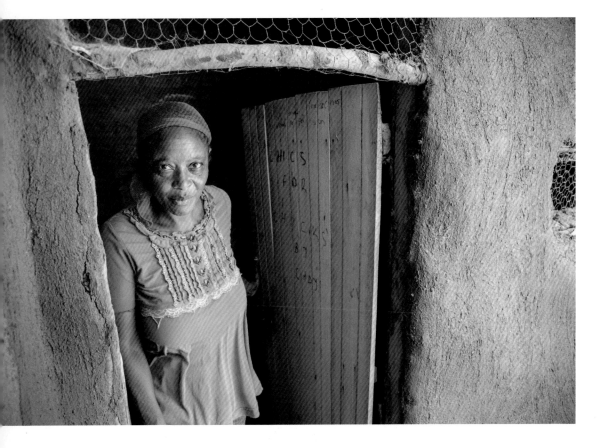

Population Health

Just days before I was to leave Eldoret, I sat down with Benjamin again, this time under a banda at the Cool Stream Restaurant near the Sosiani River on the edge of the MTRH campus. The restaurant is yet another AMPATH project. The cooks, servers, and cleaners are all HIV-positive clients of the program. Cool Stream provides them with jobs. Hundreds of the hospital's staff eat their lunches there. It has hosted farewell parties for my IU and Moi students, and I held many interviews there while researching this book.

Benjamin bought me a mango juice and ordered a passion fruit juice for himself—both freshly squeezed. He then patiently explained the AMPATH structure under Population Health. Clinical care for HIV clients is now under AMPATH Plus and is headed by Sylvester Kimaiyo. The funding for that still comes mostly from PEPFAR and so is restricted to HIV care. Population Health is made up of three "pillars," or priorities: (1) a seamless care system from primary to tertiary facilities; (2) community groups to improve health and wealth; and (3) universal health insurance. The operation was headed by the field directors: Dr. Jeramiah Laktabai, the deputy chief of party to Kimaiyo, and Laura Ruhl who lived in Eldoret full time.

I listened as Benjamin described what he oversaw in the hierarchies under these pillars. I knew many of the folks he was talking about. Dr. Matt Turissini was the AMPATH Consortium's co-coordinator of AMPATH's population health work focused on creating an accessible healthcare system. He is also Laura's husband. Mr. Cleophas Wanyonyi Chesoli was the associate program manager for Safety Net, which is somewhere under the pillar of improving health and wealth, and so was overseeing folks like Papa Anyara. And Benjamin was the program manager and focused on working with the Ministry of Health to encourage Kenyans to enroll in the NHIF. The population health plan is brilliantly described in a 2018 article in the journal *Globalization and Health* that was jointly authored by Laura, Cleophas, Benjamin, Kimaiyo, Laktabai, Bob, Adrian, and five others. I have referenced it dozens of times while researching and writing this book. I am still not sure I understand the new structures, but I am not sure it matters since everything is in transition.

As Benjamin put it, "We are spilling it over a bit." This is what AMPATH has always been very good at—spilling it over. When one part of the organization needs help, another part provides it. There is an organic, "we're all in this together" spirit that animates every project, every program, and every effort. The goal is always to get things

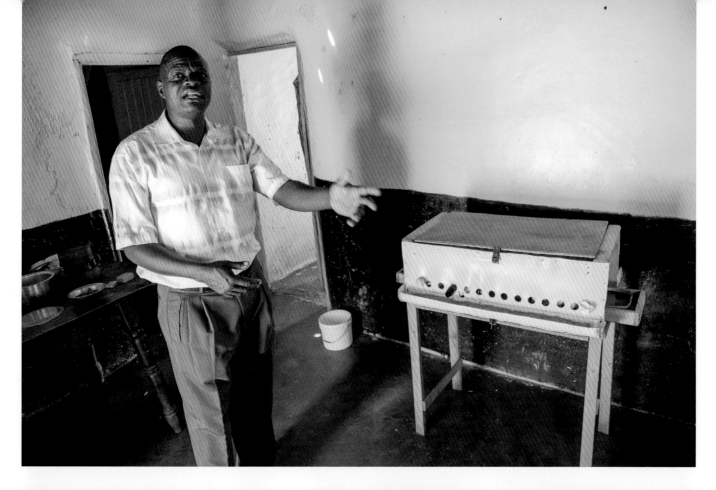

Papa speaks with Ebby in her living room. Because Ebby worked with Papa for so long, she had sufficient expertise to raise eggs into "peeps" in a brooding box in her living room, where they were safe from predators. Once the chicks were vaccinated and healthy, she supplied them to members of the GISHE group she oversaw, who used them to start their own businesses.

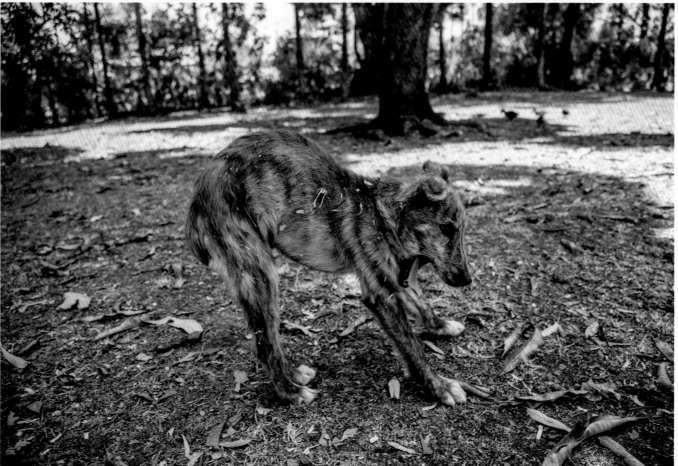

Dogs are raised to guard livestock, not as pets.

53

done instead of keeping things within the lines of hierarchy and structure.

Joe Mamlin told me a story about building the clinic in Turbo where he and Papa have met with clients since its construction in 2008 and where Ebby first received antiretroviral drugs. Joe said the leadership had located money for repairing an existing structure, but it could not be used to build a new facility. Joe and the staff at the Turbo hospital asked some local folks to build an African-style hut on the site using a few bricks and local materials. And there it was, a building that needed repair. They had money for that. Once the Turbo clinic was up and producing exceptional health outcomes, the funders were pleased that their money was well spent. It had spilled over a bit.

Back at Cool Stream, Benjamin explained to me how his efforts to enroll Kenyans in NHIF required the help of people working under all three pillars. Cleophas's Safety Net is now only for AMPATH Plus and hence only for HIV-positive people. But the NHIF goal is to enroll everyone around Turbo, positive or negative. "We are finding people out there who are very poor and cannot afford to pay for NHIF. They can't even pay for their food, let alone an insurance," Benjamin said. "Cleophas and his team, including Papa and the community guys who work with GISHE groups, are helping us out."

They were helping out on the pilot program AMPATH was running out of Turbo to see if enrollment in NHIF could be grown to sustainable levels quickly. The insurance program has been in place since 1967, when it was established by the Ministry of Health, but has effectively serviced only those with formal employment supporting payroll deductions. Because as many as 80 percent of Kenyans work in the informal sector and have no steady paycheck, the insurance program has been small despite the fact that it provides free treatment at all government-run hospitals.

In December 2018, however, Kenyan president Uhuru Kenyatta declared universal health coverage a national priority in Kenya—a key part of his Big Four Agenda for national sustainable development. Under this initiative, the government of Kenya has committed to make strategic investments in health to ensure that all residents of Kenya can access the essential health services they require by 2022. The NHIF was to be expanded to include the informal sector. For just 500 shillings per month, everyone in a family could access free healthcare. If 80 percent of households paid the fee, Kenya's health system could afford to provide it.

While I was in Kenya, the government was piloting sign-up projects in four locations around the country, including one in AMPATH's catchment area near Lake Victoria. AMPATH was running its own pilot in Turbo. The government was using radio announcements and public gatherings in the communities to encourage enrollment—typical approaches that rarely generate much response because people either fail to understand how the programs work or fail to see how new programs would benefit them directly.

AMPATH's approach was instead based on the lessons they had learned over decades of community engagement and was being conducted by people like Papa who had worked from within the communities all along. They had proven themselves to the common folks and earned their respect. A good percentage of the pilot in Turbo was funded by a grant from the AbbVie Foundation, one of the dozens of organizations that have partnered with AMPATH over the years. Benjamin said that Pfizer, the pharmaceutical manufacturer, was also doing something on the project. Just as the AMPATH workers

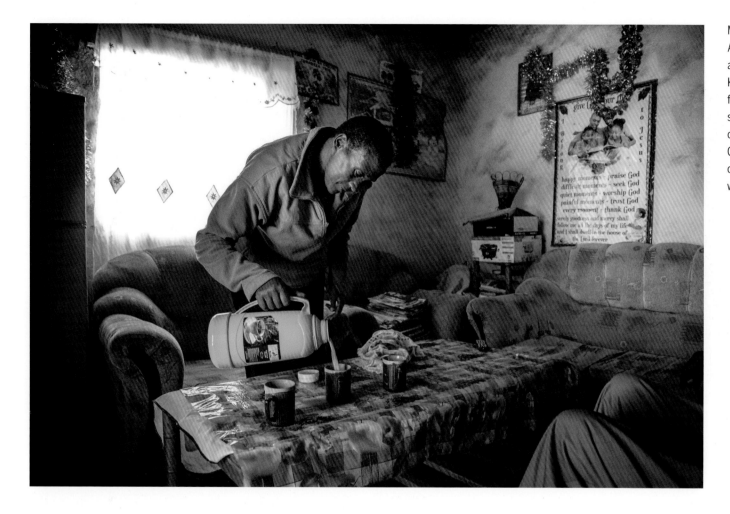

with longtime connections to the villages provided an advantage, the long-term relationships with international donors also strengthened AMPATH's efforts.

Papa trains his cadre of GESPs to talk with their GISHE groups about NHIF. He explains the benefits of enrollment and the steps to enroll. Folks in the groups trust their GESPs and feel free to ask them questions. Once they understand the benefits, they use their savings to build enrollment. "It only takes twenty shillings a day to pay for NHIF," Papa told me. Breaking it down to that small number persuades many that they can save the amount necessary. Members of the group then talk with family, friends, and neighbors who are not in the GISHE about NHIF. These conversations are supplemented with visits to their homes by health liaison officers employed by AMPATH—local people from the areas around Turbo who speak the same language and understand the local conditions.

Benjamin said,

We are hoping that our pilot in Turbo becomes universal healthcare for the country. The Kenyan government chose four areas for its pilot, but not Usain Gishu [the county where both Turbo and Eldoret are located]. We decided that the government simply offering a service was not enough. If you only look for people who can pay, a large segment of the population will be left out. We need a mechanism to help those who can only pay half or want to pay but cannot. We want everyone included. Right now, our healthcare is very selective. Those who are rich can afford to get the care, but those who cannot are suffering. Papa is an AMPATH Plus employee, but Cleophas has given us part of his time to work with Population Health.

"Population health can be the future of AMPATH," he continued. "When AMPATH started, there were no good structures to support a healthcare crisis, but now there are. AMPATH created them along with MTRH and Moi University. That relationship is great now. We can build upon the strength that we have built over the last two decades. Population health is the model. It goes beyond donor support and uses NHIF to create sustainable, universal healthcare."

Benjamin—like everyone else at AMPATH, MTRH, and Moi's medical school—understands that donor support is needed to get the program on its feet but recognizes that Kenyans must fund their own healthcare system. He is excited that NHIF represents an opportunity to move beyond a healthcare system that responds to emergency to one that focuses on prevention.

"Right now, the national healthcare budget goes to curative efforts," he said. "It could be going towards preventive measures if NHIF covered care." He went on to explain that "people like Papa are integral because they are working in our pilot area and because of the skills and knowledge that he has. He has acquired that over many years of AMPATH innovations, engaging directly with the community."

Currently, the community-level healthcare centers are functional, but people paying for insurance will expect them to be of higher quality. "Someone who has paid their NHIF must find that things are working. If not, if the X-ray is not working, if there are no drugs, he goes home and says, 'Why pay for no service?' If we're going to succeed, it has to be in partnership with the existing system. Pillar two, the health delivery team, has to make certain that what I'm promising under pillar three is real," he concluded. It has to be a coordinated effort. It has to spill over.

Still Making Change

Working with the rural poor is hard. Even seemingly small changes mean great risk for people living at subsistence level. Failure means hunger. Trying out an innovation that fails means children do not go to school or go hungry. Change is fraught, but nevertheless rewarding, as Papa explained.

I am able to change the lifestyles of the community members by training them on GISHE and agriculture. Most of them have really changed. For example, you'll find some of the ladies who have been renting are now staying on their own parcels. Number two, through GISHE, most of the members are able to pay school fees for their daughters and sons. Number three, most of them have registered with National Hospital Insurance fund. That is a success story that for me, I feel good, because through me somebody has moved a step. Through GISHE groups and through trainings in agriculture, people are now able to have food on their table. They are now able to have money in their pockets. I am motivated to do this. I am motivated by their success and to continue serving our clientele and the community at large. When the community improves, the economy of Kenya also improves. Uhuru Kenyatta cannot rule a country that is poor. Though he doesn't know it, we on the ground, we are doing something. I feel when I am doing something, the country is also doing well. The country is the communities. The country cannot work without strong communities, and the communities cannot work without a strong country.

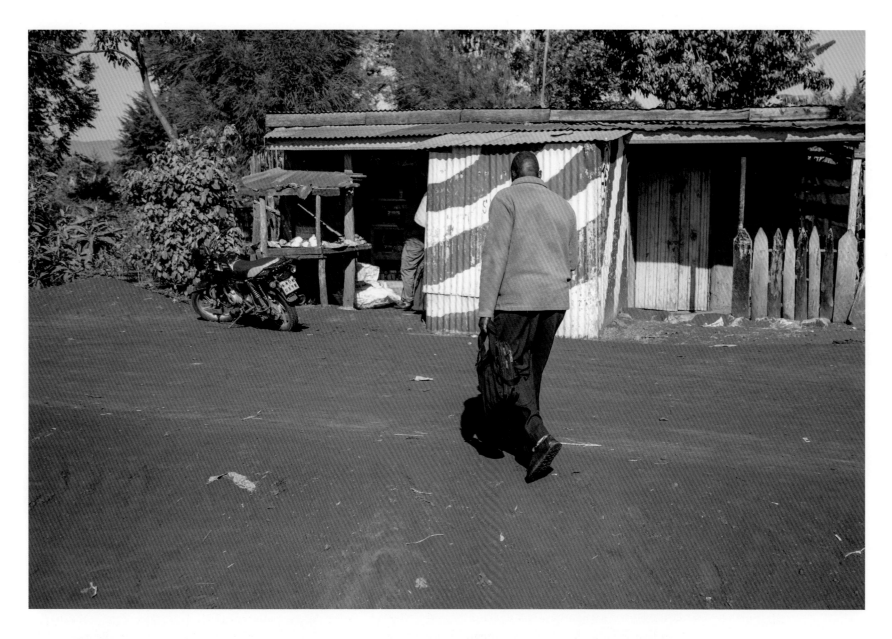

I said to Papa, "Maybe in a few years, I'll be back, and you'll be here." And he said, "I will be here, or I hope so. In AMPATH we are working on contract so I never know. Maybe the contract after December. . . . But I hope that after December, we will still be here." Papa is still there and is still making change.

Papa finishes his meeting with Marian on the day following the first rain of the "long-rains" rainy season in late April. Most of his travel is by motorcycle on the red-dirt roads of the rural area fifty miles southeast of Mount Elgon, in what Kenyans refer to as the country's breadbasket.

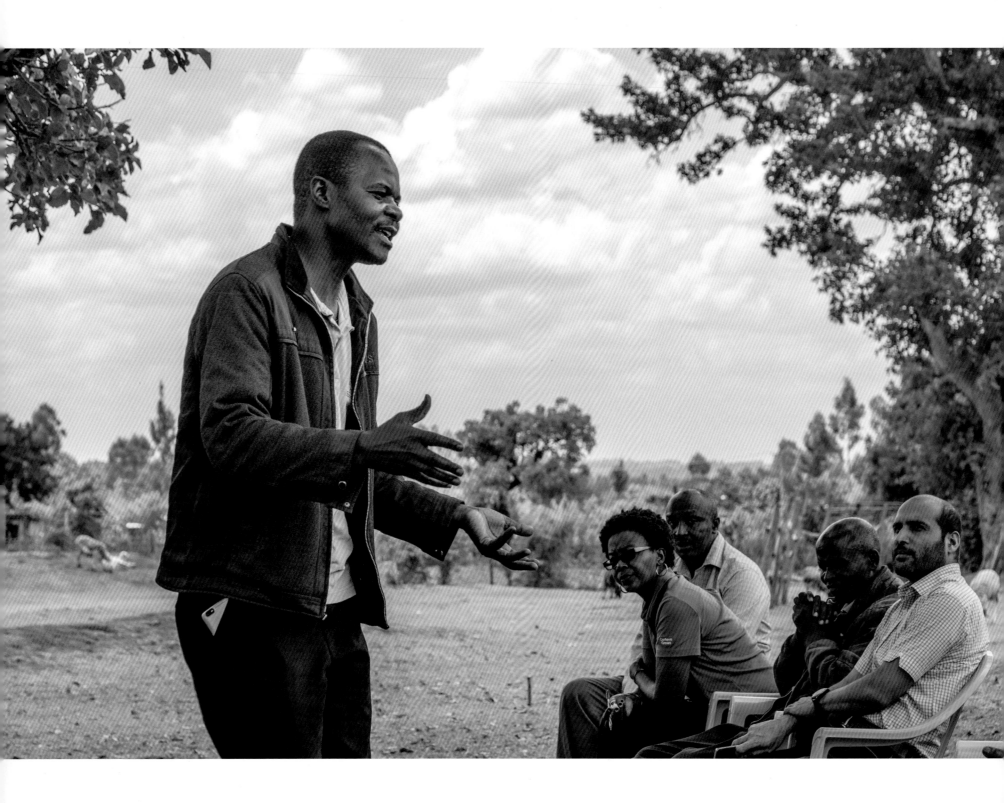

CHAPTER FIVE

Public-Private Partnerships

Kenneth and Mustafa Share Their Agricultural Expertise

For decades after Kenya gained its independence in 1963, a government job was one of the few certain paths to personal economic success. A government job provided a regular paycheck, health insurance, and financial stability that the private sector generally could not. Once you got a government job, you could relax.

The colonial British authorities had established little in the way of public services in Kenya beyond police and courts. Their schools were private, their hospitals were private, and their universities were private too. And, of course, they were available only to whites. When the British left, the new Kenyan government had to organize new institutions quickly and did so through government power and funding. Today, the public sector of Kenya includes the central government, county governments, and public corporations. It continues to provide basic goods and services that either are not or cannot be provided efficiently by the private sector at this point in the country's development. The private sector is growing rapidly, but the government still employs the vast majority of the country's teachers, doctors, nurses, and other service professionals.

Kenneth Is from Near Kitale

From 1998 to 2005, Mr. Kenneth Kisuya Malaba had one of those coveted government jobs. He was an agriculture and biology teacher at A.I.C. Chebisaas High School, a government-funded secondary school in Eldoret. Chebisaas is one of the best schools in the region. Unlike in

Facing, Kenneth Malaba has been teaching area farmers how to practice scientific methods that increase yields and strengthen communities since he joined AMPATH a decade ago. In 2019, he and his team partnered with Mustafa Ghulam (far right), a visiting expert from Pakistan, on a fellowship sponsored by Corteva, a longtime partner with AMPATH.

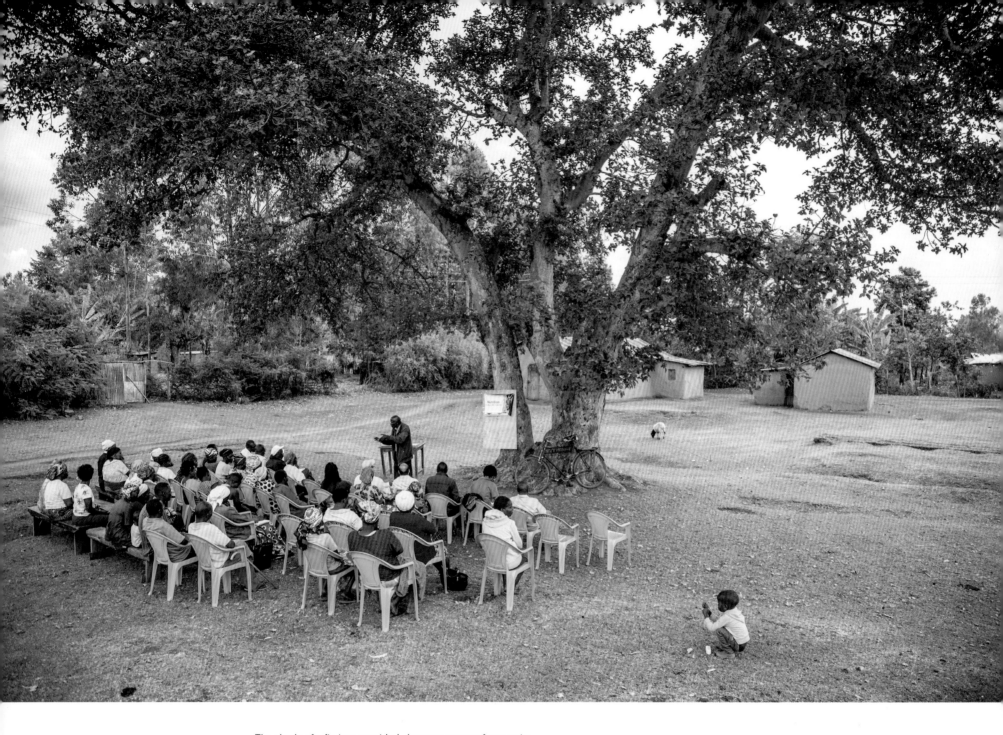

The shade of a fig tree provided classroom space for county livestock officer Sampson Araka, who began the workshop by explaining to members of the Kaptweti Olgay Dairy Co-operative that while their farming practices had proven reliable over generations, the modern scientific methods presented by Mustafa from Pakistan could improve their operations dramatically.

the US, it is the government schools that attract the best students in Kenya. Those who do not make the cut attend privately funded schools.

When Kenneth was there, Chebisaas's sixty-nine-acre campus on the outskirts of Eldoret sat next to another one hundred acres where the school's staff raised 60 dairy cows and 500 chickens, plus vegetables and maize (corn) for the boarding school's dining hall. Kenneth was in charge of all that too. He had earned his bachelor's degree in agriculture and proven himself as a capable teacher and farmer. He was all set and could have relaxed in his government job.

But he was restless and wanted to do more to help the farmers on small plots of land he had lived among as a boy in Bungoma County, close to Mount Elgon. In 2006, Benjamin Andama and Cleophas Chesoli, heads of the FPI, asked him to join the team as an agriculture expert. Kenneth said yes. He later wrote his master's thesis about food security among the socially and economically vulnerable smallholder farmers of western Kenya and publish his research in an academic journal (Malaba, Otuya, and Saina 2008).

"I left government so I could join AMPATH. It was a new experience altogether. People kept saying, 'Your background is agriculture. How come you are getting into the health sector?'" he told me as we sat in the middle seat of a van on our way to a seminar for farmers just outside Kitale. Kitale is Kenneth's working area. It is about forty-five miles north of Eldoret and sits in the shadow of Mount Elgon, an extinct volcano that lies on the border with Uganda. "The exciting thing was that I was going to continue on with my career in agriculture, but now I would ensure that our clients and smallholder farmers were food secure and income secure," he said. "I had never worked in a health environment before, so it was quite challenging. In fact, I almost resigned during the first

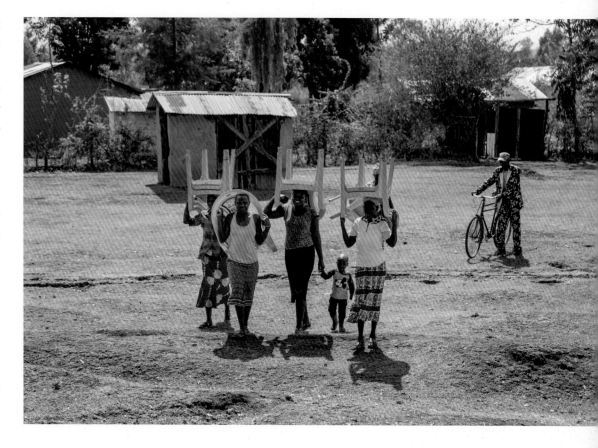

month because the AIDS epidemic was so terrible. The way those clients were coming to us. They were extremely vulnerable, dying on the benches outside the clinic. It was so scary."

At that time AMPATH was treating nearly fifty thousand HIV-positive clients, but more than two million Kenyans had contracted the virus, and tens of thousands were newly exhibiting symptoms of AIDS every year. "So, I say, 'Is this the place I am going to work?'" he recalled. "But soon I began liking my work and carrying out interventions and seeing that these people could recover. I liked that I could empower them economically. Food security issues—that became my motivation. I liked that I could see people getting back on their feet and getting back to their economic livelihoods."

Several members of the co-op had attended their GISHE group on the other side of the open field and carried their chairs to use at the Corteva workshop. Others borrowed benches from the nearby church.

Within AMPATH's treatment area, 70 percent of the population depends on agriculture for both basic nutrition and economic security. Kenneth currently works with a small team, called Safety Net, that includes Cleophas, Mr. Donald Cheminingwa, and Ms. Pamela Busieney. It is essentially a continuation of the FPI but within AMPATH's all-encompassing population health plan. Over the years, they have helped area farmers organize themselves into cooperatives that allow them to operate shared resources, including storage facilities, animal veterinary services, and educational seminars where more than thirty thousand farmers have learned efficient farming techniques, farm management methods, and marketing plans to commercialize their products. Kenneth and his team are making a difference as AMPATH staff, often working with private partners from the West to build the infrastructure of knowledge upon which Kenya will grow economic sustainability.

Mustapha Is from Near Lahore

At about the same time Kenneth was doing his extension work with dairy farmers in Kitale, Mr. Mustafa Ghulam was working with dairy farmers just outside Lahore, Pakistan, three thousand miles from Kitale. Unlike Kenneth, Mustafa worked for a private company. He had joined Pioneer Seed in 2010 as a dairy-animal nutrition expert and was focused on the agricultural development of small farmers in the Punjab.

As Mustafa recalls, "I grew up in a small farming family back in Sangla Hill, Pakistan, near Nankana Sahib"—the most important religious site for the Sikh religion, located about sixty miles east of the city of Lahore. "I saw my father struggle with farm productivity and profitability, so I have very closely observed the challenges the small farmers face," he said. In high school he had hoped to study medicine but could not afford it, so he decided to go into agriculture studies at the university.

"It is good that I went into this profession. I got my degree in dairy nutrition and animal husbandry in 2006 and joined the Pakistan Dairy Development Company. It was a government project, but all of the experts were from New Zealand and Australia," he recalled. "They trained the dairy sector so that when they left, we had the expertise." Mustafa credits those foreign experts with much of the success of the dairy industry in Pakistan over the last decade. The country is now the third-largest milk producer in the world. "There is still a lot of development to do in dairy in Pakistan, but at least we can now say that the industry is shaping up," he concluded.

In 2018, Mustafa read of a fellowship sponsored by Corteva Agriscience, Pioneer's parent company. It had just been spun off from DowDuPont to become the largest standalone agricultural organization in the world. The Corteva Grows Food Security fellow would spend six months in Eldoret, and Mustafa was interested. Corteva's predecessor, Dow AgroSciences, had been partnering with AMPATH since 2013. Every six months it sent a new agricultural expert to Eldoret to help AMPATH's own development team.

I talked with Mustafa about his fellowship as we sat in the living room of Hilltop House, a ten-bedroom home just across the street from where I was living in the IU House neighborhood. All the Dow AgroSciences experts had lived there. Indeed, Hilltop was where most of AMPATH's long-term visitors stay: nurses, med students, researchers, and others working in Eldoret for more than a few weeks, including my fellow Fulbrighter, Dr. Kyle Carpenter, who lived there for a year. "When the fellowship was announced, I studied the dairy industry in Kenya and found lots of similarities between Pakistan and Kenya," Mustafa said. "I thought, this is a good opportunity to

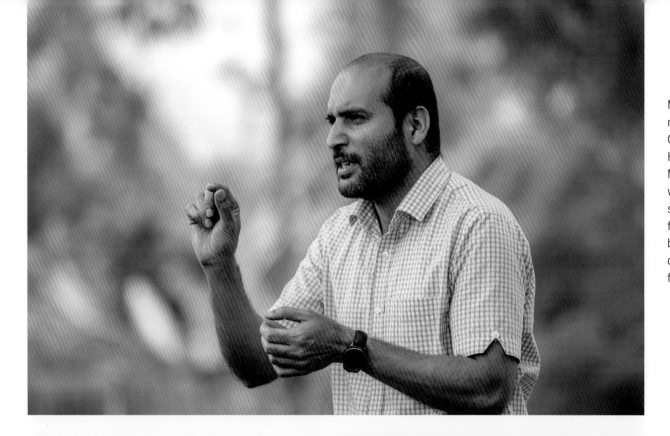

Mustapha Ghulam spent six months in Kenya as a Corteva Grows Food Security fellow. He partnered with Kenneth Malaba to organize workshops where he could demonstrate scientific practices for dairy farming using silage to better withstand periods of drought and increase yield for small-plot farmers.

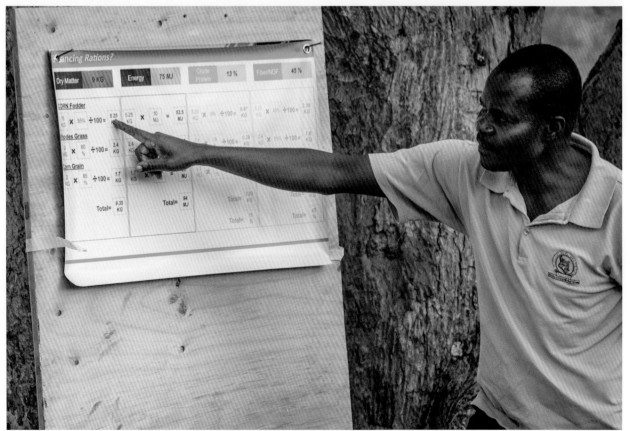

With no facility for PowerPoint, the team printed their slides on large sheets for display during the presentation; the sheets were then left for the co-op to use for their own purposes.

Right and below, Work in the fields was slow for the farmers around Kitali because the rainy season was late to arrive in 2019. Most of these farmers own one to five cows on as little as a quarter acre of land. They cooperatively share facilities like grain storage bins, grazing lots, and veterinary structures. Kitale is just thirty miles east of Mount Elgon, an extinct volcano straddling the Kenya-Uganda border.

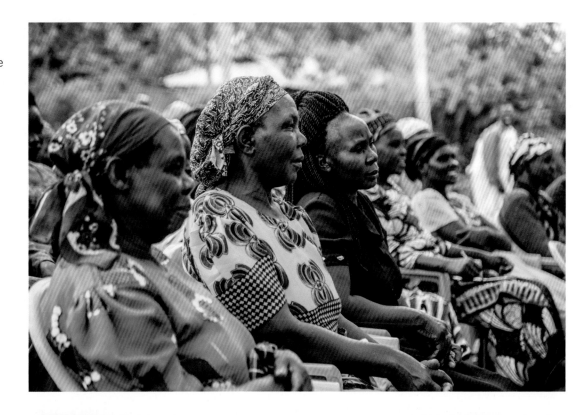

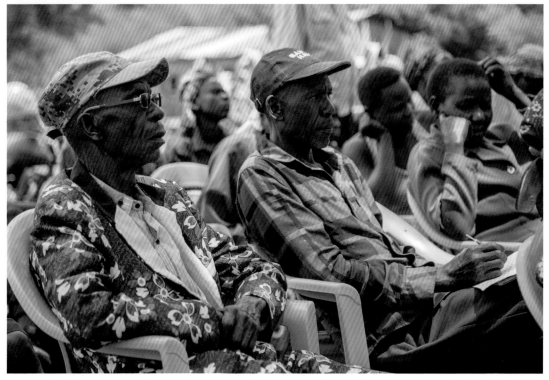

share the successes we have achieved. I thought the models we used could work here as well. Their productivity and profitably could be enhanced. I had learned much from the New Zealand and Australian experts, so I thought now is the time for me to pay back to society for what I have learned."

Mustafa had spent years working at Pioneer to increase dairy production through the use of silage—green fodder like corn stalks that have been compacted and thereby preserved by acidification achieved through fermentation. The process reduces spoilage, extends storage life, and enhances nutritional value. "Farmers told previous fellows that they needed help increasing the productivity of dairy animals," he said. Nearly every farmer in the region has a cow for milk. "Because I have dairy nutrition experience and agronomic training, I could help them keep their animals more profitably." Farmers also told the fellows that the differences in yield between wet and dry seasons caused difficulty, so Mustafa proposed educating Kenyans with small farms about silage that could be preserved from the rainy season and provide needed fodder during the dry season when field grasses are sparse.

"Most people working for Corteva in Kenya are commercial or research agents, but the first thing we are told when we come here [on fellowship] is to take off our commercial hat. 'You are going for philanthropic purposes,'" he said. To drive home the point, he said fellows often work with crops Corteva doesn't even sell seeds for, like onions, tomatoes, and potatoes—crops that are essential for Kenyan farmers.

"You have seen that map—health and wealth," Mustafa said, referring to the diagram that guides AMPATH's efforts toward population health (see image later in the chapter). "If you want to improve the health of the people, especially the rural poor, I would say then you have to improve the wealth of the people. Their bread and butter

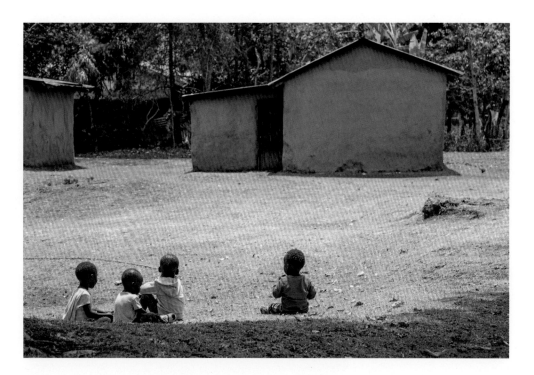

is farming, and there are two benefits to improving this. For good health, they need good nutrition. And secondly, if they have money, they can purchase NHIF."

Earlier in my career, I had traveled to Pakistan a half dozen times to put on workshops that trained the country's journalists on techniques for reporting on social issues. I developed many close friendships there and have hosted four postdoctoral fellows from Pakistan who did research with me in the United States. I therefore particularly enjoyed talking with Mustafa. He was the first non-American Corteva fellow. Perhaps because a sizable and influential portion of Kenya's citizens trace their ancestry back to South Asia, the local farmers seemed somehow more comfortable with him than with other foreign experts. Regardless, Mustafa clearly brought knowledge from the outside that was of value to the Kenyan farmers he and Kenneth worked with during the fellowship.

Children wait for their parents on the edge of the field where the workshop took place.

Mustafa works through a nutrition example while Kenneth listens. Mustafa was born to a farming family near Lahore, Pakistan, and after university worked for years with the Pakistan Dairy Development Company, a government project, where he was taught modern practices by experts from New Zealand and Australia. He said it was his privilege to pass on his expertise to the people of Kenya.

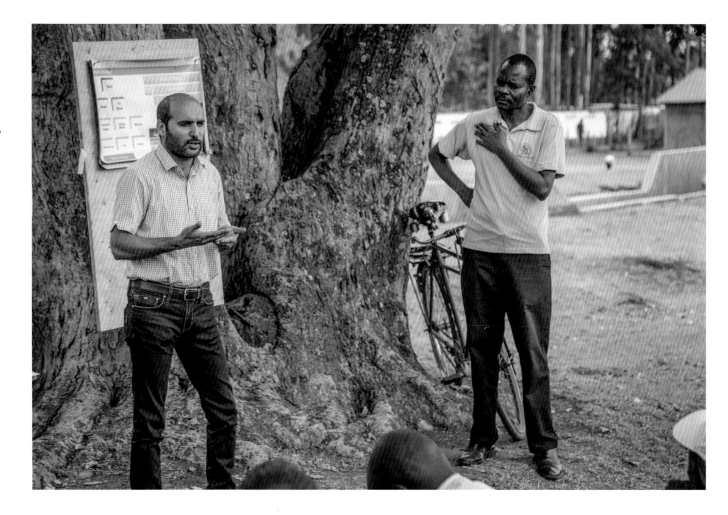

As the global climate changes, the dry seasons are getting longer and the rains less predictable. The silage and other husbandry practices Mustafa and Kenneth taught to area farmers will help them provide for their cows more consistently and efficiently. Kenya has two seasons: rainy and dry. Historically, the "long rains" came from March to the beginning of June and the "short rains" came from October to the end of November. This pattern was predictable, and the modern farming practices developed in the Great Rift Valley, first by farmers from Britain and South Africa and then by Kenyans after independence, have turned the area into the breadbasket of the country. Maize is the staple food, and it is eaten three times a day as

ugali, a thick porridge served with African vegetables and stewed meats. The drink of choice is cow's milk, and it is difficult to overestimate just how essential milk is to the local cuisine and culture. The local people were primarily herders before British occupation. Their cows provided them with necessary protein, both as milk and as blood carefully drained from the cows' necks. A mixture of the two was placed in calabash gourds to create *mursik*, a fermented milk variant with deep roots in the area's history. Though the practice of drawing blood from cattle is no longer practiced widely, fermented milk is sold in modern grocery stores, and there are even claims that *mursik* makes the Kenyan long-distance runners so fast.

From AIDS to Population Health

AMPATH and Its Partners

From the very beginning, AMPATH has encouraged private foundations and companies to join with it in public-private partnerships to develop Kenya's healthcare infrastructure. Indeed, the start of the project that would become AMPATH was underwritten by an Indianapolis philanthropist, Mr. Marty Moore. Moore was a high school history teacher in the 1980s. One of his students wrote a research paper about Dr. Ellen Einterz, a medical missionary in Nigeria. Moore met with Einterz and her brother Bob. In that meeting, he learned about the vision that Bob, Joe, Charlie Kelley, and Dave Van Reken had for global health, and he fronted the funds for them to explore a potential partnership with a medical school in Africa or Asia. The team found Mengech and Moi University and Eldoret.

Eight years later, Craig Brater, the chairman of the Department of Medicine at IU, committed $500,000 to initiate an endowment to support IU's care, training, and research mission in Kenya. Another IU School of Medicine faculty member, Dr. Dave Matthews, worked with his wife, Ms. Emily Matthews, to lead the congregation of the Second Presbyterian Church in Indianapolis in a fundraising effort that built four surgical suites at MTRH in 2000. These and other early collaborations proved that just as the partnership among Moi University, the MTRH, and Indiana University could overcome structural divides, public-private partnerships were also effective in achieving health outcomes.

But private-public partnerships really took off in a big way with the creation of the AMPATH Consortium in 2001. First there was the coalition of foundations that funded HIV treatment for HIV-positive mothers. Then, in 2003, the Purple Foundation of Canada gave a half-million-dollar "A Bridge of Hope" grant that greatly extended the ability of AMPATH to treat HIV-positive people. The

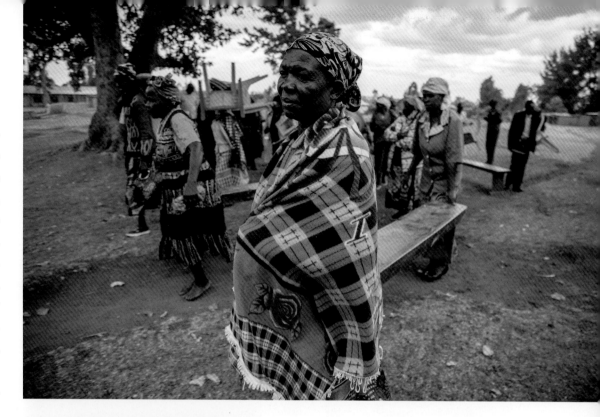

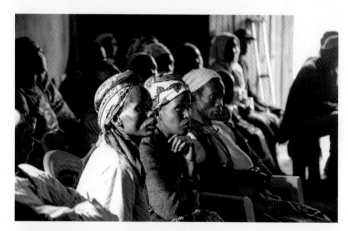

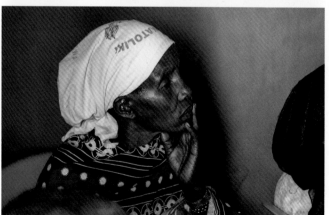

Above, Just as the AMPATH team was finishing up its lecture on animal nutrition, the highly anticipated "long rains" started to fall. Everyone moved into a church on the edge of the field that had been the classroom for the day.

Left and below, Once inside, folks listened to additional speakers from the local county extension office and asked questions of the experts who had just provided them with so much detailed information.

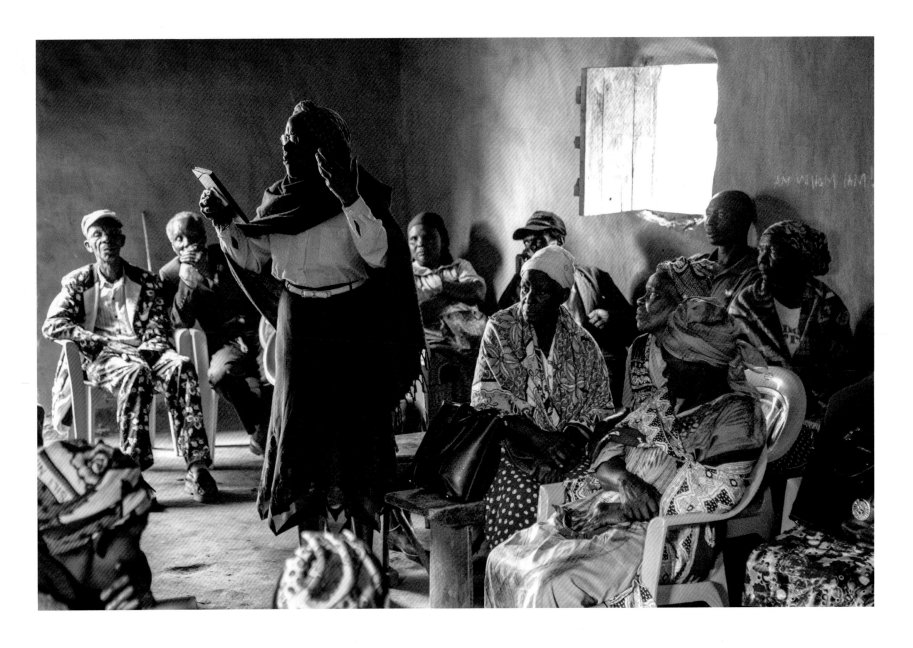

consortium landed its first PEPFAR grant of $6.5 million in 2004, followed by $60 million in 2007. PEPFAR funding has continued to sustain the campaign against HIV, but there is little doubt that these public monies and the funding provided to MTRH and Moi University by the government of Kenya over the years were predicated upon the earlier private-public partnerships AMPATH had built with foundations associated with medical and pharmaceutical companies like Eli Lilly of Indianapolis, Pfizer of New York, Abbott Laboratories of Illinois, Astra-Zeneca of Maryland, and Merck & Co. of New Jersey, as well as organizations with broader missions like the Gates Foundation of Washington, the largest private foundation in the world.

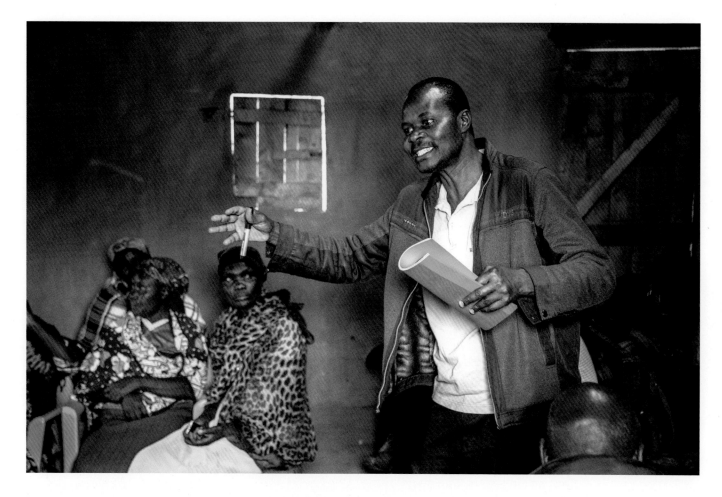

During the early years of HIV treatment, foundations and private individuals provided HIV drugs, laboratory equipment and testing technology, and funds to build major infrastructure on the MTRH campus, like the AMPATH Centre and the Riley Mother Baby Hospital, which was birthed with the help of IU's Dr. James Lemons. More recently, the Chandaria Cancer and Chronic Diseases Centre, named after Mr. Manu Chandaria, a Kenyan businessman and philanthropist who helped fund the building, represents the broadening of AMPATH's mission to address other chronic diseases. Dr. Patrick Loehrer Sr., director of the Indiana University Melvin and Bren Simon Cancer Center in Indianapolis, headed the effort to build the center and coordinated donations from the Ruth Lilly Philanthropic Foundation, Pfizer, and the Simon Center.

Increasingly, these public-private collaborations are guided by AMPATH's recently created population health model, which was described in a 2018 academic publication written by many among the leadership at AMPATH: Tim Mercer, Adrian Gardner, Benjamin Andama, Cleophas Chesoli, Dr. Astrid Christoffersen-Deb, Jonathan Dick, Robert Einterz, Nick Gray, Sylvester Kimaiyo, Jemima Kamano, Beryl Maritim, Kirk Morehead, Sonak Pastakia, Laura Ruhl, Julia Songok, and Jeremiah Laktabai. In "Leveraging the Power of Partnerships," they described how AMPATH has built powerful partnerships

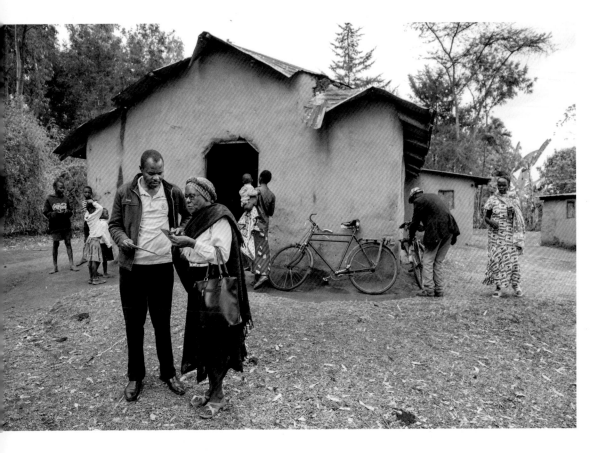

Above, Kenneth and Maurice exchange email contact information so they can follow up with each other. About sixty farmer members of the co-op attended the workshop, and Maurice was sure there would be more questions once her co-op began making plans for better nutrition management.

Facing, The Ministry of Health–AMPATH population health care delivery model's learning map.

to move beyond the traditional disease-specific silos in global health to a model focused on population health. They share how AMPATH worked with strategic planning and change management experts from the private sector to collaboratively develop a novel approach and shared vision of population health to achieve strategic alignment with key stakeholders at all levels of the public-sector health system in western Kenya.

Beryl Maritim, one of the authors and the program manager for the population health initiative, met with me during my first week in Eldoret. She explained that public-private partnerships have been essential in building capacity and supplementing the investments in healthcare made by the Kenyan government. Direct assistance from foreign governments, whether PEPFAR for HIV care

from the US or support from other global partners, cannot be expected to continue indefinitely, however. Kenya must fund its healthcare system from its own wealth. That said, foreign funding from private partners is expected to increase, particularly for research, since MTRH and Moi University now provide such a well-managed and collaborative operation.

Beryl explained how AMPATH had partnered with private-sector strategic planning and change management experts on a "learning map" that provides a visualization of population health that key stakeholders at all levels of the public-sector health system can use to understand and contribute to the future of healthcare in western Kenya. Under this model, the healthcare system is presented as a constructed pipe that waters the tree of health and wealth for the family. The pipe sits on the strength of the lessons and best practices in providing care, such as training next-generation leaders in healthcare, research, and innovation over the course of several decades of collaboration between AMPATH and the MoH. The ministry's role is represented by the bigger figures at the top because of their importance in the scalability and economic sustainability of population health efforts countrywide. The smaller-scale but numerous MoH and AMPATH programs produce the inputs that fill the pipe in coordination with others.

Beryl has explained the map to dozens of people since its development. "When participants like Ministry of Health understand the map, their buy-in and goodwill to champion these efforts is greater. Likewise, when donors understand it, their contributions are more targeted, effective, and responsive to the actual needs on the ground," she said.

> If you have a donor supporting oncology, they come here, they understand the map and maybe at the end they would consider providing additional funding to support

From AIDS to Population Health

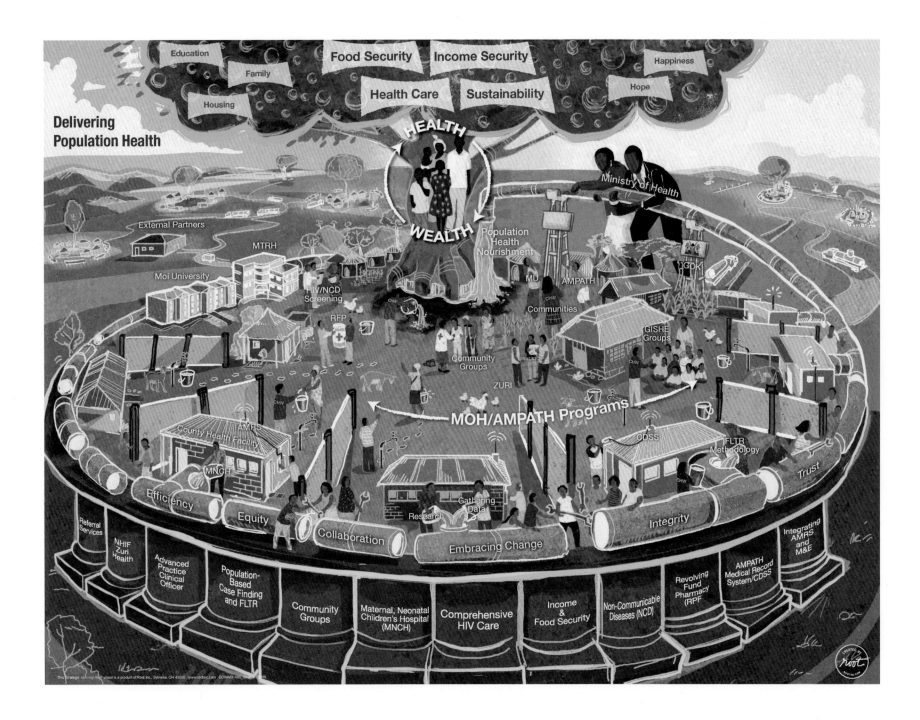

Delivering Population Health

more than just oncology. They come to appreciate that the patient is part of a developing health system that is working to provide comprehensive coverage where it did not exist before. . . . There are two audiences for the map.

Participants in Kenya gain an understanding of how well it has been thought out in its comprehensiveness. Donors see that too and see how necessary it is that their focused contributions contribute to the overall goals. At the end of the day, this must be a homegrown project. External partners play a crucial role, but ultimately the success of the initiative depends upon Kenyans building a self-sustaining system.

Training Farmers in the Shade of a Fig Tree

It was a Wednesday morning in late March when Mr. Francis Dagala pulled the van Mustafa had hired into the district hospital parking grounds in Kitale. We had picked up Pamela and Donald an hour earlier in Eldoret and were now meeting Kenneth at his office before heading out to where the Kaptweti Olgay Dairy Co-op held its meetings. The first of five workshops Mustafa and Kenneth had planned for the co-op would take place shortly under a giant fig tree in the middle of a field just off a dirt road maybe five kilometers from the hospital.

No one was there when we arrived, so the team began setting up by nailing a piece of plywood to the fig tree at about eye level. When workshops are held in town, they meet in a hotel and use PowerPoint, but there was no screen, no projector, and not even walls at this location. Instead, the leaders had printed the instructional materials on yard-wide sheets that hung on pegs. Changing the slide was a simple matter of removing the top sheet to reveal the next. This idea had come from Pakistan via Mustafa, and the AMPATH team thought it was great.

A few moments later, dozens of farmers came around the bend carrying plastic chairs above their heads. They had been at their regularly scheduled GISHE meeting and quickly settled down under the big tree and to wait for the presentation. Others joined the initial group, and soon there were about sixty farmers ready to learn how to increase the yield of their cows.

Joining the presenters was the county livestock officer, Mr. Sampson Araka, a local man who already had the trust of those in the crowd. After Kenneth welcomed all to the workshop, Sampson took the floor and said, "This is the first time I have seen AMPATH come out to help us with cows." He said people in Kitale had always had a good relationship with AMPATH and the staff who worked on HIV, and then mentioned that he was excited to hear AMPATH's presentation on farming.

Kenneth and Mustafa next took turns explaining the material: a description of a cow's digestive system, the ideal housing for dairy cows, various feed types, the storage requirements for silage, and chart after chart of complex formulas for determining when to feed, what to feed, and for how long. The farmers took notes and frequently took photos of the presentation slides with their mobile phones.

One older couple commented on the complexity of the information being presented and asked if perhaps there were shortcuts. Mustafa and Kenneth explained that correct proportions of feed and water are critical and dependent upon the specifics of individual cows and particular inputs. They explained that while calculation of the components and formulas was a bit daunting, this knowledge was the key to increasing production. They were teaching agricultural science to people who may not have finished high school but certainly knew how to raise cows by traditional methods.

And then, just as they were reaching the final slide, it started to rain. The rains were about two weeks late at that point in March. The lessons presented promised a way to better survive this type of drought, so nobody left. Instead, they picked up their chairs and benches and moved into the nearby church, where their questions could be answered by the experts. Once inside the small tin-roofed building, Ms. Jane Omutsani, the co-op's director, began asking specific questions about the lessons. Others joined in, often asking in Swahili that was translated for Mustafa by Kenneth. The two experts took turns answering until everyone was satisfied.

Sampson then took the floor again and talked to folks with the passion one expects to hear from a preacher rather than a government agent. He spoke at some length in Swahili and then concluded in English, "I don't know how long AMPATH will come around, but I know that if you learn these lessons today, you will have a good system for taking care of your animals and your family." He urged the farmers to attend all the workshops and bring others to the next one. Kenneth then concluded the meeting by saying that Mustafa would soon go back to Pakistan but his lessons would "remain forever if you use your mind and heart."

Paying Back

Back at Hilltop that evening, I asked Mustafa why he would leave his family and spend six months all by himself in a country so far from his own. He said, "I feel it is the responsibility of every professional, not only in the agriculture sector, but also medical, pharmacy, or communication, that whatever he gains from society he must give the same back to society. I have gone away from my family for six months to repay what I have been given."

"Paying back" for one's opportunities is a common refrain around the IU House. The folks who live in Hilltop often arrive out of a sense of obligation, but, like Mustafa, they come to understand that they also have much to learn. "I am gaining new knowledge and new solutions," he said. "I am gaining cultural knowledge and learning new things that I can take back when I return to Pakistan." Good partnerships benefit both sides.

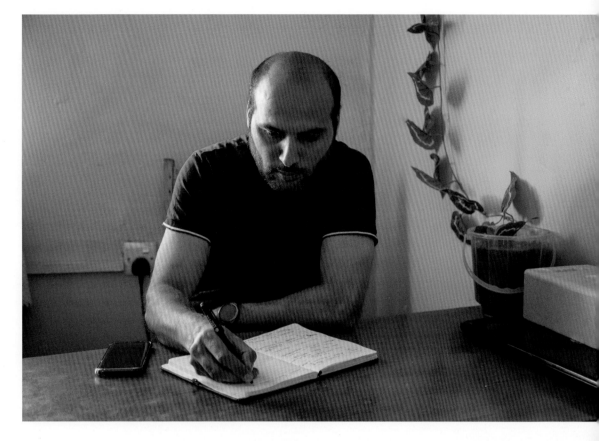

As he prepared to leave Eldoret and return home to his family in Pakistan, Mustafa said, "I feel it is the responsibility of every professional, not only in the agriculture sector, but also medical, pharmacy, or communication, that whatever he gains from society he must give the same back to society. I have gone away from my family for six months to repay what I have been given."

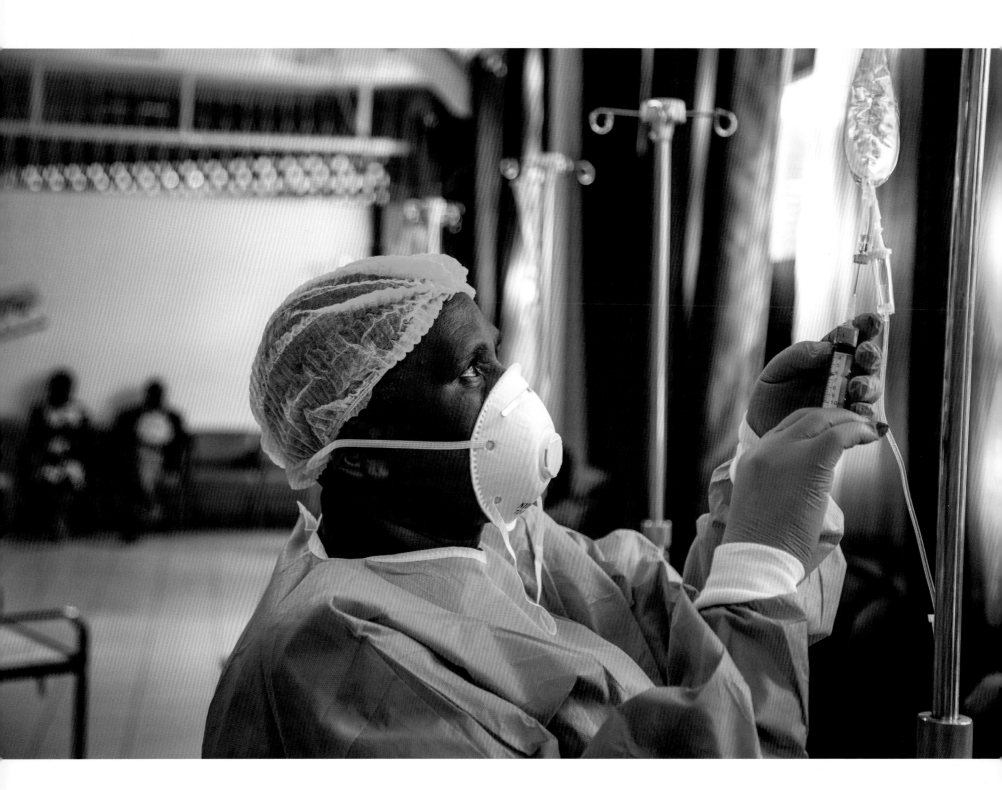

CHAPTER SIX

Managing Chronic Diseases

Pamela Were and Her Colleagues Are Making Cancer Survivable

I waited for Ms. Pamela Were to take a break as I sat in the only unoccupied chair in her Chandaria Centre office suite across the hall from the hematology lab. She sat less than two feet from me in one of eight tiny cubicles, each just big enough for a small desk and chair. She was typing emails on the desktop computer while answering frequent calls on her Apple iPhone and Samsung Galaxy mobile phones. From time to time, she would tap her Apple watch, sometimes to silence the ringing iPhone and other times just to check her schedule. Every five or ten minutes, someone would come by to ask a question or to give a report.

Pamela was a senior nurse practitioner and the outreach coordinator for AMPATH Hematology and Oncology. Back in 2006, she delivered a paper at the World Cancer Congress conference in Washington, DC (Were et al. 2006). Today it remains uncommon for women from the developing world to deliver papers at international conferences, but it was rarer still then. Pamela, however, is one unusual woman. In that first conference paper she described a pilot program AMPATH had been running in four remote clinics to screen for early detection of cancer and administer chemotherapy to those diagnosed with Kaposi's sarcoma, a type of cancer common in HIV-positive patients. In just eight months, they had identified three hundred people in the early stages of cancer—early enough that proper treatment would likely save their lives.

Contrast this against the typical identification of cancer at the time. Patients would present at the MTRH with very advanced stages of the disease, making care difficult,

Facing, Pamela Were, a senior nurse practitioner, prepares fluids for a patient in the Chemotherapy Administration Area of the Chandaria Cancer and Chronic Diseases Centre on the MTRH campus in Eldoret. They treat thirty to sixty patients per day.

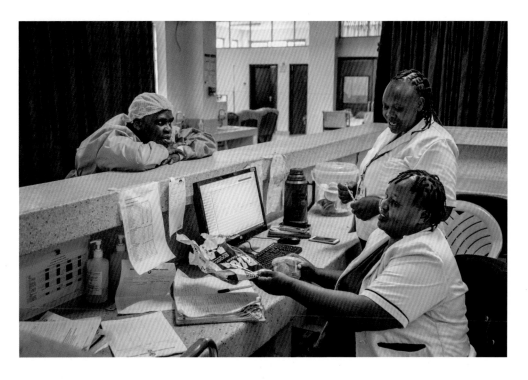

expensive, and ultimately unaffordable due to the patients' low socioeconomic status. The only option was palliative care to manage their impending death and attendant pain.

Cancer is a chronic disease, as are cardiovascular diseases, diabetes, blood diseases, gastric ulcer, and lung diseases. Together, they account for 70 percent of global deaths and are the leading drivers of morbidity, mortality, and disability globally. They disproportionately affect lower-income countries like Kenya where healthcare infrastructure is still developing (Allen et al. 2017). Pamela's paper demonstrated that early detection of cancer was possible in rural Kenya, but it was best done at the village level, not at the tertiary care facility in Eldoret. When Pamela's paper was published, the appropriate infrastructure was not in place to screen for cancer in remote clinics. But when I met her, she was working with a team delivering on the promise described in that academic paper. AMPATH outreach clinics take place every two or three weeks now, and they make a difference in the lives of thousands.

Road Trip to Lake Victoria

The sun was still below the horizon when the van picked me up from the IU House. Pamela welcomed me and introduced me to Ryan, the driver. She said we would next pick up Drs. Nicholas Kisilu and Chris Mwaniki, both

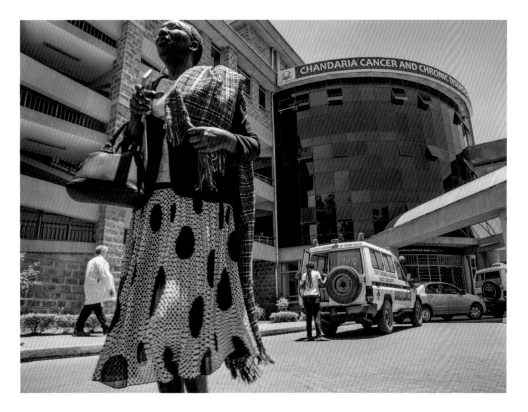

Top, Pamela chats with Margaret Fwamba, principal nursing officer, and Judy Koech, nurse in charge, about the day's workflow and some nice sesame seed cakes that a friend of Margaret's made for the staff.

Left, The creation of the Chandaria Centre was spearheaded by Patrick Loehrer Sr., director of the Indiana University Melvin and Bren Simon Cancer Center in Indianapolis, and was completed in 2015.

From AIDS to Population Health

physicians at the AMPATH Oncology Institute, and then Mr. Stephen Kiptoo, the project coordinator, before setting off on the six-hour drive to Sori, a village of nine thousand on the eastern edge of Lake Victoria. As we sat in a gas station parking lot, Pamela led us in prayer.

As is so often the case in Kenya, we arrived at our final destination much later than I had expected. Along the way we took a two-hour detour through Kisumu, the country's third-largest city, to pick up medical supplies needed by the clinic at the Sori Lakeside Hospital the next day. A small boy carried the cardboard box of supplies out to us from a cluster of small buildings as we waited by the side of the busy highway. Two hours later it was six in the evening and getting dark. We had only made it to Homa Bay, an hour away from the lake, but the van was needed back in Kisumu, where the fifth member of the team had spent the day. Ryan would bring Dr. Fredrick Chite Asirwa, director of oncology at the MTRH, to the hospital in Sori the next morning.

Pamela called Mr. John Okeyo, the hospital director, and he sent his hospital's ambulance to collect us and take us on the final leg of our journey. Chris and I were the tallest, so we got the front seat with the driver. Pamela, Nicholas, and Steven crowded into the back, and we set off in the dark. No one likes to drive late at night in Kenya. The driver drove with the ambulance's lights flashing and the sirens on. As we cruised through the cool night air, Chris told me about a trip he had taken a few years earlier to Indiana. An expert in sickle cell anemia, Chris had visited clinics in Nappanee and Shipshewana in the northeastern part of the state, where the Amish people have high rates of blood diseases. He liked the Amish, admired their religious commitment, and was impressed by the extensive care they receive for their rare bloodborne illnesses.

Then we hit a dog as it crossed the road. We three watched as it happened, but there was nothing to be done.

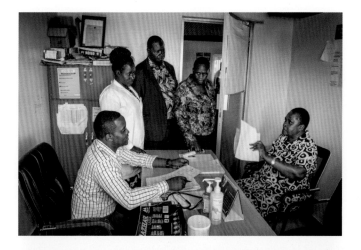

Nicolas Kisilu talks to Jasinta Ochido, who returned to hear the results of biopsies taken two weeks earlier, as Pamela and John Okeyo, the hospital's director, listen. Both tests were negative. Jasinta said, "We fear because we don't have money. Because it [the clinic] was free, I decided to come. Now I have the news we prayed for. My children are aware, and I am happy."

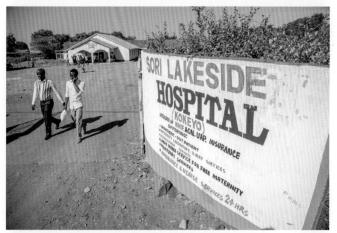

Sori Lakeside Hospital is privately owned but partners with AMPATH to provide free screening sessions to all who arrive and register. The hospital accepts NHIF insurance and refers clients to government-run clinics for treatment.

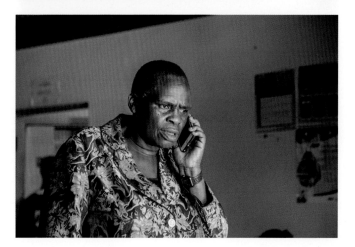

Pamela confirms details of her colleague Chite Asirwa's arrival for a cancer screening clinic at a hospital on the shore of Lake Victoria, about 150 miles from Eldoret. As the outreach coordinator for AMPATH Hematology and Oncology, she organized dozens of screenings every year.

Animals are killed on the road rather frequently in rural Kenya. Had it been a goat, it would have legally belonged to us, and we could have taken it home for our own use. But we were looking for cancer, not meat. We didn't say much more until we checked into our lakeside hotel in Sori. It was nearly nine at night. The clinic would start at eight the next morning.

Hands That Make the Pain Go Away

Pamela had told me of road trips she made many times much earlier in her career. She had started working at MTRH when it was still just a district hospital in 1987. She spent a year on the labor ward before being moved to the oncology ward.

But before joining the big district hospital, she worked at a provincial hospital in Nakuru in the gynecology ward. Nakuru then was roughly the same size as Eldoret and is the halfway point for those traveling by car from Eldoret to Nairobi, the nation's capital and largest city. Pamela was seeing a lot of advanced cancers of the cervix. "Most staff tended to ignore them," she said, "but somehow, I found a rapport with them."

There was no treatment available for these patients in Nakuru other than painkillers. Most of the staff would inject patients with saline solution because the process of administering painkilling drugs was tedious. Soon the patients would be crying again from the pain. Pamela didn't find this practice acceptable or ethical, so she would give pethidine, the only available painkiller, even though it required far more effort. She recalled, "This made the patient identify with me, and they would say, 'I want to be injected by that sister. She uses her hands so it makes the pain go away.'"

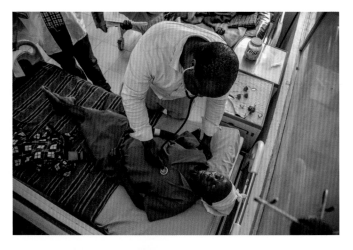

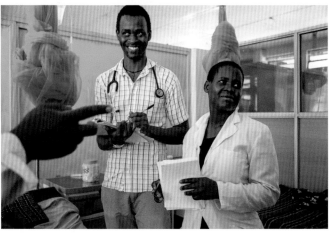

Top, Chite conducted clinical rounds on the wards with the hospital's staff and examined seventy-one-year-old Deborah Akeyo Acharo. She had been admitted to the hospital because of a failing heart but was additionally diagnosed with cancer. Chite spoke with Elisha, and together they determined that her continuing care should be outpatient. Additionally, Chite recommended Deborah be sent to hospice, where palliative care could be provided, and promised to put Elisha in touch with a hospice near Eldoret. The annual incidence of cancer in Kenya is about thirty-seven thousand new cases with an annual mortality of twenty-eight thousand cases.

Bottom, Doctor Faustin Obbo Otin and Clinical Officer Millicent Amolo.

But the pain never fully went away, and most patients died for lack of treatment because advanced cancer of the cervix could only be managed by palliative radiotherapy. A few, however, would be referred to the Kenyatta National Hospital in Nairobi, the nation's oldest hospital and, at the time, the only hospital with radiotherapy. Pamela took them there, but the journey was maddeningly difficult every time.

She said, "I would have eight women going with me to Nairobi. The ambulance would escort us up to the stage"—the escarpment on the edge of the Great Rift Valley that was still eighty miles from the hospital. Those final miles had to be in a *matatu*, the sixteen-passenger minivans that serve as public transportation throughout the region. "With only half of the van full, the driver would not go. Some bad drivers would tell me to get out with those 'stinking ladies.'"

Advanced cervical cancer creates a foul-smelling vaginal discharge that cannot be cleansed away with normal hygienic care. Eight women in such condition would have made a small van quite unpalatable to most drivers and passengers. Pamela would search the taxi park for a driver willing to take half a load to the hospital. Sometimes it would take hours to find such a kind soul.

By the time they reached the hospital, it would be mid-morning, and the women had been traveling all night. "The sun was warm. The flies were all awake. With the discharges they had, when they walked with you, the flies would follow. People in the street were running away, but I would still go with them," she said.

Pamela and her patients would arrive at the referral desk hoping for help from the radiologists. "But the minute I would get there they would say, 'Whoa! Those are Nakuru patients. They stink like Nakuru patients.' They

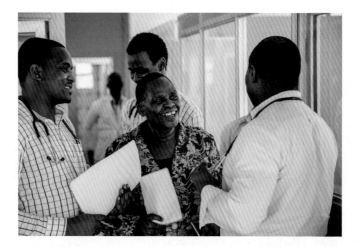

Nicolas and Pamela laugh at a joke Chite made.

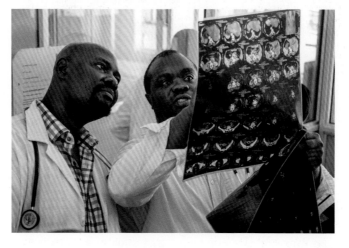

Elisha and Chite confirm a diagnosis.

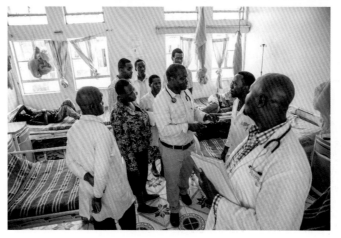

All the AMPATH and Sori Lakeside staff joining Chite on rounds listen as he consults with Chris Mwaniki about treatment for a patient with sickle cell disease. The disease has contributed significantly to the mortality rate in children younger than five, primarily because of late diagnosis, educational gaps among service providers, and lack of access to appropriate treatment.

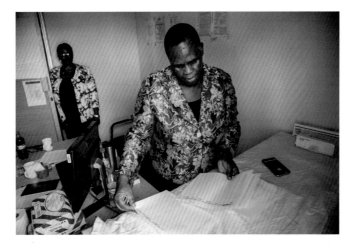 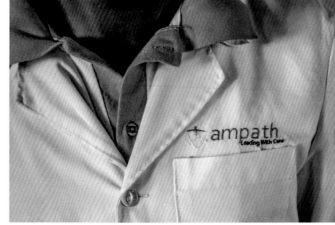

would say, 'This one you take back, this one you take back,' and sometimes I would end up coming back with all of the patients," she said. None got any care, and the journey back to Nakuru felt even longer. She concluded, "Inside myself I would ask, 'What can I do to make a difference? These people are dying a very painful death, but what can I do?'"

Sori Screenings Start at Eight

The outreach clinic in Sori was to begin at eight in the morning. We arrived at about nine and, according to "Africa time," were a bit early. Chite was already there, however, and settled into the small room where he would meet with patients the rest of the day. Okeyo, the hospital director, and his assistant, Mrs. Betty Obiero, had organized the staff into a support network for the outreach clinic. Two clerks at a table on the front porch were registering the folks just beginning to arrive. Most were here to get the results from tests for breast or cervical cancer that had been taken two weeks earlier. All had been assigned an AMPATH patient number, and all would forever be in the digital medical record system that has formed the backbone of care going back to the earliest days of the

IU-Kenya Partnership. They might ordinarily pay for services at the Sori hospital, but as AMPATH clients, their screenings and the result consultations were free.

Most patients arrived on *boda boda*, the ubiquitous motorcycle taxis that ply the streets of villages and towns throughout the region and charge only a few shillings per ride. A few came in automobiles, but many more walked in from homes as far as five miles away.

Sori Lakeside Hospital is a private hospital. Public health facilities in the region range from the referral hospital in Eldoret, where AMPATH is headquartered, to district hospitals with dozens of doctors, like the one in Kisumu, to subcounty hospitals like the one in Homa Bay that might have four or five doctors, down to village-level dispensaries likely staffed with little more than a clinician and a nurse. The public system is funded by the government and is generally recognized as inadequate. Privately owned clinics and hospitals serve the third of the country that has private insurance and is therefore able to pay for services. The two systems exist side by side but do not often formally interact. Chris explained to me that Sori Lakeside was the only facility in the area that had adequate facilities to support AMPATH's mass screenings. The screenings would overwhelm the nearby public

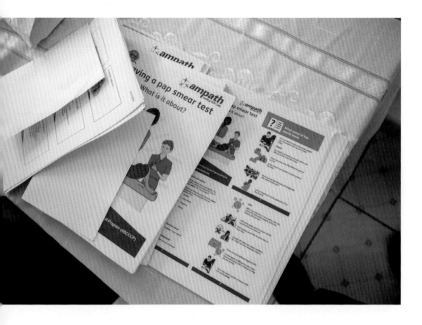

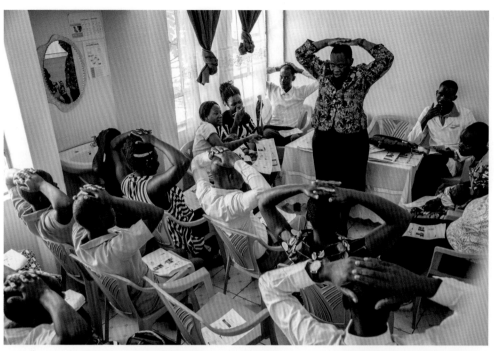

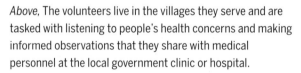

Above, The volunteers live in the villages they serve and are tasked with listening to people's health concerns and making informed observations that they share with medical personnel at the local government clinic or hospital.

Top and bottom right, Pamela instructs a class of community health volunteers on how to conduct a breast examination as Stephen Kiptoo, the project manager (far right), listens.

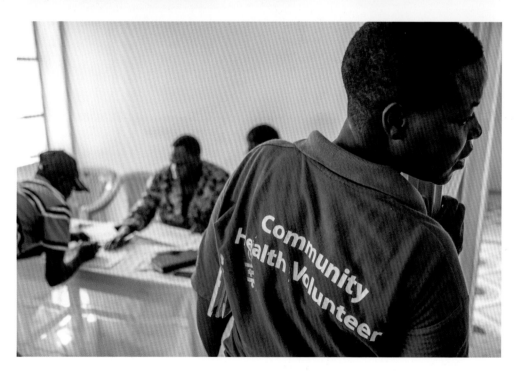

dispensary, so Sori Lakeside hosts the outreach clinics because the director John Okeyo wants his neighbors to have access to the free care. He and his son, Dr. Elisha Onyango Okeyo, understand that early detection means treatment will be possible, whether at their hospital or elsewhere. Like Pamela, they too have seen late-stage cancers with no hope of cure. The outreach clinic provides the hope people around Sori need.

By lunchtime, Pamela and her colleagues had delivered results from the previous clinic to more than one hundred people. Some were relieved that the tests were negative, but many more would leave knowing they

In the United States, the disease primarily affects African Americans, and a similar 1 percent of their babies are born with the disease. But when a vaccine protecting against invasive pneumococcal disease was introduced in 2000, the US saw sickle cell–related death among children younger than four fell by nearly half. The vaccination rate in Kenya is still low because few parents know they have the trait and fewer know their child has the disease. Early detection is therefore critically important. By the end of the day, Chris had screened 130 children, identified nearly 100 who were positive, and referred all of them to the hospital for treatment and possibly vaccination.

Community Health Workers

While the medical staff were delivering results and doing screenings, Betty assembled about twenty community health workers (CHW) in a seminar room near the back of the hospital. Pamela and Steven held a training session on how the CHWs should instruct their clients on breast self-examination. These folks work for little or even no pay but nevertheless form a strategic link between medical personnel at county hospitals and ordinary people in their villages. They often alert people that they may have early stages of cancer and encourage them to seek care at public facilities. Their work at early detection is critically important if Kenya is to reduce incidents of terminal cancer.

After her training session with the CHWs, Pamela joined Chite as he went on ward rounds with Elisha and other staff who seldom have contact with a physician of Chite's expertise. Elisha is one of two of John's sons who work as clinicians at their father's hospital. While out on the wards, Chite examined seventy-one-year-old Ms. Deborah Akeyo Acharo. She had just been diagnosed with cancer, although she had been admitted to the hospital because of a failing heart. Chite spoke with Elisha, and

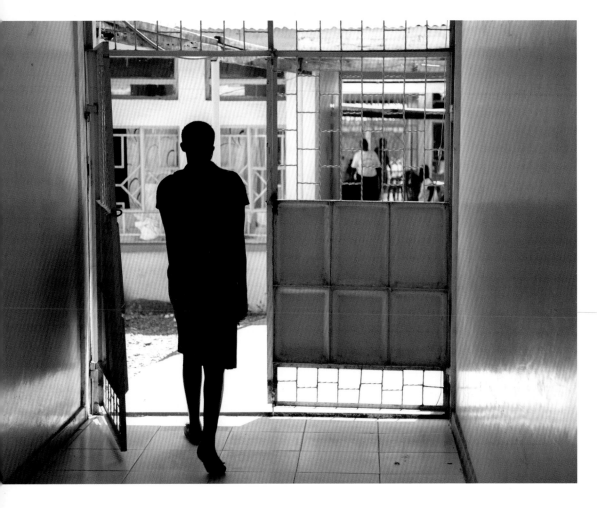

A patient walks from one ward to the next. Sori Lakeside, like most hospitals in Kenya, is composed of many small buildings with covered walkways connecting them, allowing air and light to circulate.

had cancer in their bodies. For most, the diagnosis was early enough that treatment and remedy were possible. They left with referrals to the local public hospital. The team was also screening for sickle cell disease. Chris had screened sixty children so far, all of whom were positive.

In sub-Saharan Africa, about 1 percent of all births (perhaps 240,000) are affected by sickle cell disease, an inherited blood disorder that deforms the red blood cells. Depending on the region, 50 to 90 percent of children born with sickle cell disease die before they reach their fifth birthday. The condition causes 6 to 15 percent of all deaths in children younger than five (Uyoga et al. 2019).

together they determined that her continuing care should be outpatient. Indeed, Chite recommended she be sent to hospice, where palliative care could be provided. But it was Pamela who delivered the news to her because, of the four caregivers in the room, she was the only one who spoke the woman's local language. Pamela had grown up in Sori and was therefore speaking to someone from her own tribe. Deborah was also HIV positive, but because of her consistent adherence to the antiviral drug regimen she had been on since testing positive decades earlier, her viral load was undetectable and not a concern for her cancer treatment.

The team's policy is to see every patient who comes to the outreach clinic. At five in the evening, we travelers from Eldoret were in the van and ready to call it a day—except, of course, for Pamela, who was finishing up with Betty. I myself was dog tired, and all I had done was lug around a couple cameras and observe these professionals working with the nearly three hundred people who had come to the clinic that day. I could only imagine how draining it must have been on the AMPATH team—delivering good and bad news, screening people worried they had cancer, and telling parents their child had sickle cell disease. I could see on their faces that they were exhausted but nevertheless pleased by the good work they had accomplished.

And then a middle-aged man walked up to the open van door and asked me if the clinic was still open. I looked back at Chite for an answer. He climbed out of the back seat and escorted the man inside the hospital. We waited another twenty minutes before Pamela and Chite returned to our van. We still had that six-hour drive home. Darkness was setting in as quickly as it always does near the equator and always at six thirty, all year round. Sunset and sunrise are the only truly dependable appointment times in Kenya.

She Could Have Gone Anywhere

When I interviewed Pamela in the Chandaria Centre and she told me about those early days of her career, when she would travel to Nairobi with patients and return to Nakuru with little to show for it, I asked her why she didn't just leave. She has presented two dozen papers at international conferences. She had a diploma from a university in Great Britain. She had done fellowships in Australia, Canada, and the United States. Her credentials and expertise would make her very attractive to any number of hospitals in the developed world, where medical resources were plentiful and salaries far larger. She said,

> What I realized is that whenever I do placement abroad, I see places where patients are fewer than the people taking care of them. The people who have the skills that I went to learn are more plentiful than the patients they are caring for. When I return home, it is clear that the people who have those skills are less than the patients they are caring for. My services are of more value when I bring them back home than were I to add them where there are enough professionals. That is what really motivates me. I serve a person who would otherwise not have anyone to help them if I did not come back.

A Long, Dark Ride Back Home

Chite was with Pamela, Chris, Nicholas, Kiptoo, and me in the back of the van on the return trip from Sori to Eldoret. The outreach team was relaxed, and they talked freely about their day, enjoying a sense of shared accomplishment. Discussion of the day's work was animated by laughter. Everyone told funny stories about their youth, life in their villages, and previous outreach clinics in places far from Sori and Eldoret. These were people who knew each other very well, traveling across a countryside they had visited frequently together. By

Bernard Odkicipbo tidies a room near the MTRH. A free screening at Sori Lakeside Hospital in early March showed he had cancer. Because each treatment takes many hours, patients traveling long distances to Eldoret cannot be processed and treated in the same day. A grant from Takeda Pharmaceuticals provided him a place to stay the night just a few minutes' walk from the Chandaria Centre.

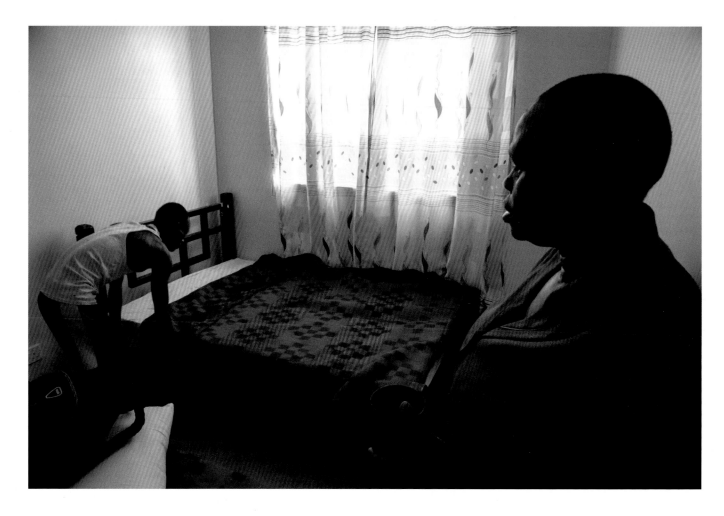

about midway, possibly as we were crossing the equator, the laughter slipped into the dark humor medical personnel sometimes revel in. Their jokes and stories would have sounded morbid and tasteless to almost anyone outside our van, but it sounded therapeutic to me. They talked of death and dying, of pain and suffering, and they laughed in the face of it all. Research shows that this sort of humor is more common among the highly intelligent (see Willinger et al. 2017), and there was no doubt in my mind that this van was packed full of intelligent people. They were under stress as they treated patients with advanced-stage cancers—cancers that should have been caught early on when treatment was possible—and that stress catches up

with a body. These friends found mutual release and acceptance in the black humor they had given into that dark night. Just as they turn the pain of others into the care of AMPATH, so they turn their grief over the suffering they see into a humor that provides relief and comfort and camaraderie. It was laughter of love for their patients, for each other, and for good medicine.

There was another outreach clinic the following week in Meru on the other side of Mount Kenya—an eight-hour drive from Eldoret. The team again screened all who came. And then they returned two weeks later to deliver the results and screen for sickle cell. There will be another outreach clinic a couple of weeks later over on the border

From AIDS to Population Health

with Uganda or maybe near Lake Baringo. Each clinic, whether held in a government hospital, a private hospital, or one of AMPATH's clinics, will identify dozens or even hundreds of new cases of cancer. Each of those patients will meet with nurses and clinicians in the following weeks. Some will be sent to the MTRH in Eldoret for chemotherapy or radiation treatment in the Chandaria Centre.

Pamela will be there. She will be answering calls on her mobile phones in the little cubicle office. She will help nurses in the treatment areas locate needed drugs when the hospital pharmacy is out. She will laugh and joke with the nursing staff and comfort the patients as they sit in the overstuffed chairs as chemicals drain into their arms to kill the cancer in their bodies. Some will be HIV positive, but that doesn't really matter anymore. AMPATH has enough free drugs for all now, and the virus that was once a death sentence is now just another chronic disease the country's healthcare system is working to detect early and treat effectively. The patients who make their way from villages that hosted an outreach clinic may well spend twice or even three times as much time making the journey from their village to Eldoret. Most will travel with thirteen other Kenyans in a minivan that may make thirty or forty stops between a place like Sori and Eldoret. They will arrive tired and lonely and in need of care. Pamela and her team will be there.

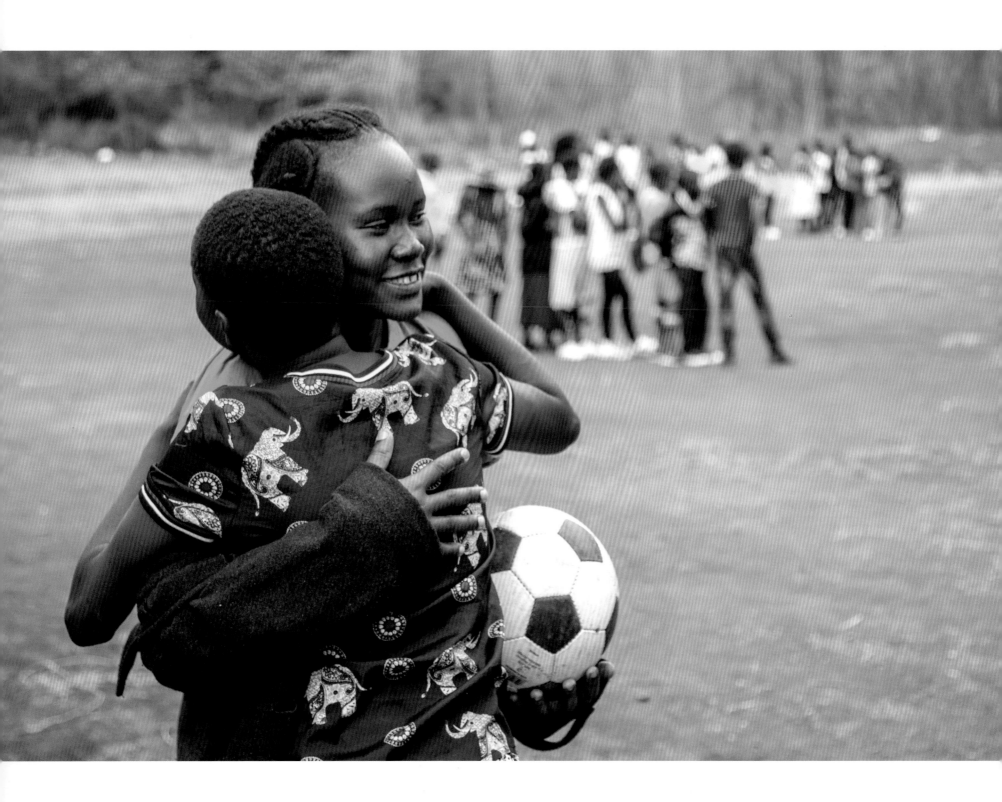

CHAPTER SEVEN

Rafiki Centre for Adolescent Health

A Clinic of Their Own Where Young People Help Heal Themselves

Mr. Brian Sang Kipchumba has always been HIV positive. When he was born in 1995, there were no antiretroviral drugs to prevent a mother from transmitting the virus during childbirth. Positive women delivered positive babies—whether they knew it or not. Most babies died within the first year. Most of those who survived the first year still undiagnosed died of AIDS-related illnesses as children.

Brian was among a very small number who lived a dozen years in the chronic, asymptomatic stage before being tested, diagnosed, and put on a regimen of drugs to keep his viral count low and his body strong. AMPATH had started when he was six years old, and by the time he was nearing the end of primary school, its home testing and counseling (HTC) project was going out into communities all over western Kenya. One team arrived in Brian's school to test everyone twelve years and older. Brian was thirteen. He tested positive.

A team member met with Brian and his parents in their home to deliver the result and discuss treatment. "My mom was confused by my result," Brian said. She had never been tested and had not shown any symptoms of AIDS. Nevertheless, a test confirmed that she too was positive and most likely had had the virus in her body since before Brian was born.

I met Brian during Rafiki Fun Day in April 2019. It was the last Friday of break for students of all levels—primary to university. More than 170 had registered for the day of games and fellowship that would take place at the Rafiki Centre for Excellence in Adolescent Health located

Facing, Judy Odiwa, a volunteer social worker at the MTRH Rafiki Centre for Excellence in Adolescent Health, leads a confidence-building exercise on the hospital's graduation ground during Rafiki Centre Fun Day in April 2019.

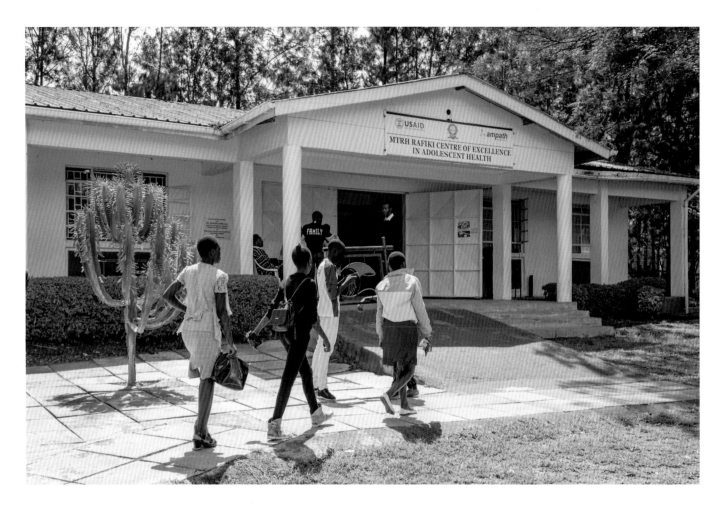

close to the huge graduation grounds on the edge of the MTRH campus. Brian was a peer counselor at Rafiki and was ready to enjoy his final Fun Day as a client of the comprehensive care clinic (CCC) assigned specifically for youths. In a couple months, when he turned twenty-four, his medical files would be moved to an adult-care CCC in the MTRH.

As a teenager, Brian had struggled with disclosure of his HIV status. Every month he visited the CCC known as Module 4 in the big AMPATH Centre building on Nandi Road, right in the middle of the MTRH campus. I asked him about those days as we stood near a big boulder in the Rafiki Centre's garden as preparations for Fun Day

were getting underway. He explained to me that Module 4 was for children only. While Brian knew his status, many of the others there did not. Like him, they visited once a month for checkups and to have their ARV prescriptions filled at the pharmacy. But Brian also met weekly with a support group of youths about his age who did know their status and were struggling to understand what it meant. It was there that Brian met Sarah Ellen Mamlin.

Sarah Ellen and her husband, Joe, had lived in Eldoret for a year in 1992 as IU team leaders. When she returned eight years later, she was distressed to find children wandering the halls of the MTRH's pediatric ward with little to do. Many of those children were there because their

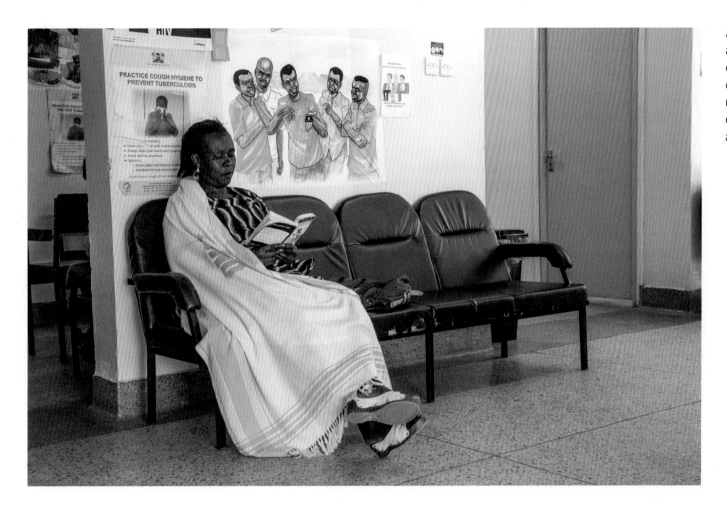

A mother waits for her child's appointment to conclude outside the clinician's office on a cool January morning. Posters remind clients to practice safe sex and respect each other.

mothers were sick with AIDS. Others were themselves sick. Backed with a generous gift from Ms. Sarah (Sally) Test of Indianapolis, Sarah Ellen persuaded administrators to rebuild a space in the MTRH where children could go to play and dance and learn while they or their family members were in the hospital. Sarah Ellen and pediatric nurses like Ms. Patricia Buretto organized MTRH staff and volunteers to help the children cope with the trauma of a long-term visit to the hospital. Patricia and Sarah Ellen soon realized that the older children needed psychological care and began working directly with Module 4.

Brian learned about the Sally Test Centre from Sarah Ellen and spent time there in 2009 as a volunteer helping with the younger children. At the same time, he was taking a leadership role in his support group and thinking deeply about the psychological needs of youth. He understood that the children in the center would soon need mental care as well as physical care. It was as if Brian was being trained for service at the future Rafiki Centre.

Stigma and CCCs

The Rafiki Centre space is dedicated to the unique needs of youth, including those living with HIV. CCC Modules 1, 2, and 3 in the AMPATH Centre provide treatment and support for HIV-positive adults, and Module 4 provides

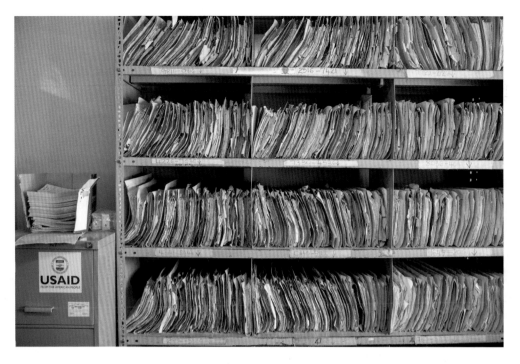

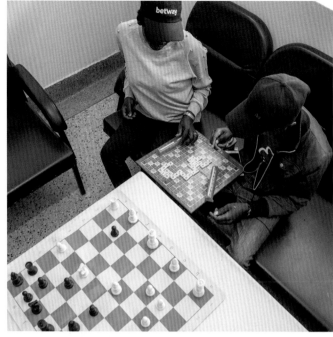

similar care for positive children. Dozens of other CCCs are located at county and subcounty hospitals around the region served by AMPATH, and they have provided services for tens of thousands since their establishment in the early 2000s. Rather than simply providing diagnoses and ARVs, the CCCs also screen for cancer, hypertension, malaria, diabetes, and a host of other chronic diseases. Comprehensive means that clients get all the medical care they need or are referred to other facilities in the Ministry of Health system.

But they were not quite comprehensive enough for patients between ten and twenty-four years of age. Kenyans refer to this age group as "youths." The range may seem wide, but it captures children facing challenges most ten-year-olds do not know as well as twenty-three-year-olds who are still struggling with lives that include HIV. Rafiki provides these youth with treatment, nutritional support, peer support groups, educational sessions, and more, all within a facility that is physically distant from the hospital buildings they visited as children. In Swahili, *rafiki* means "friend," but I was repeatedly told that, in this case, it also means "home."

The Rafiki Centre started up in 2016, and Brian was nicely prepared to mentor his peers in the group and individual sessions that are so critically important to gaining the trust of incoming clients. He had struggled with the stigma of being HIV positive but came to accept his status with the help of counselors. "It is still there, but it has decreased by a very big percentage. I first had to learn to understand 'self-stigma,'" he explained. The stigma people with HIV encounter from other people is obviously problematic and reasonably well known. But less evident to the general public is that positive people often blame themselves and internalize the stigma.

According to a recent study by Pantelic and colleagues (2017), internalized HIV stigma occurs when a positive person internalizes perceived negative public attitudes toward people living with HIV and accepts them

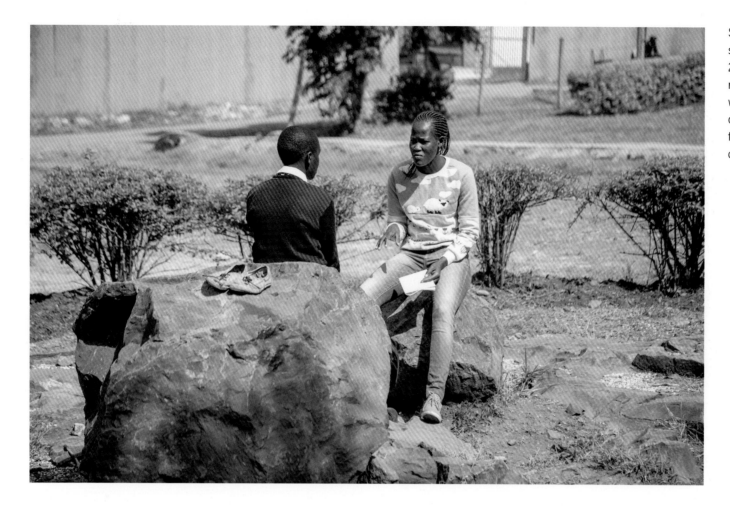

Susan Rono, a peer mentor since Rafiki opened in 2016, likes to sit on the big rocks in the center's garden when she talks with new clients. "We can be away from the others and they can be relaxed," she said.

as applicable to themselves. By evoking strong feelings of shame and worthlessness, internalized stigma can pose a serious threat to long-term physical and mental health. "It is what's said behind your back, the avoided glance, the assumed dislike, that leads positive people to pull away and isolate themselves" (Cairns 2013, 1).

Brian said the counseling sessions organized by Sarah Ellen in Module 4 had helped him find comfort and caused him to feel less alone. He said the Rafiki Centre provides many opportunities for HIV-positive adolescents to "just be alone to discuss how we feel without being threatened. . . . With peers you can be open. They know." He said that in a peer group you can admit that,

"hey, I forgot my pills this week and didn't have them at school." Others in the group have probably done the same and can share what happened. "It's never as bad as you think. People make mistakes, and it is not the end." This is the Rafiki approach: "We are friends here."

Bongo Flava

When I arrived at eight in the morning on Rafiki Centre Fun Day in late April, a stereo was set up on the veranda, and two young guys were playing bongo flava music by Tanzanian Diamond Platnumz. I had to ask who he was. The guys were happy to tell me because they didn't figure

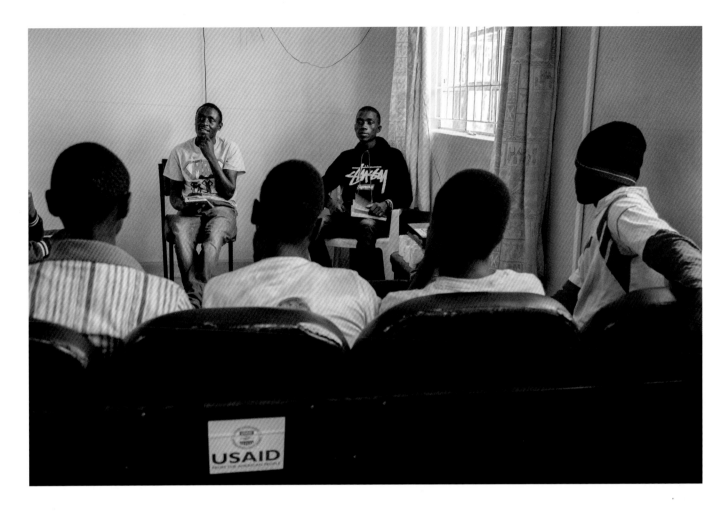

Peer mentors Hillary Kiptoo and Gideon Kemboi lead a group support session in a room that also serves as the social room and the salsa dance studio.

an old *mzungu* would know anything about modern music. Telling the story of AMPATH had been hard from the start since I am not a Kenyan and it is very much a Kenyan story. Now I was trying to bridge both cultural and generational differences. I was trying to understand young people who were dealing with myriad health crises that are incredibly personal in nature. I had been dropping by the center every couple of weeks for four months. I knew the staff pretty well, but their clients remained largely unknown to me. All of the youth were welcoming and kind. They chatted with me amiably, but none showed any interest in opening up to a stranger. The magic of Rafiki is that they do indeed open up *to each other*.

A pair of wide metal doors were opened wide, and about seventy-five people ages fourteen to twenty-four sat on chairs tightly crammed together in the reception area. Center staff welcomed them: the manager, Ms. Jane Chemon; the clinician, Mr. Archie Shume; the triage nurse, Ms. Judy Butu; and the retention officer, Ms. Ann Jeptoo Tallam. Everyone in the crowd was either a client or a friend of a client. Parents looked in from the veranda, and since I had agreed not to photograph the clients, I stepped outside to chat with the folks closer to my own age.

Earlier in my visit, when I was just learning about Rafiki, Sharon Chemtai, the public relations officer for AMPATH Plus, had explained Rafiki's relationship to the

From AIDS to Population Health

larger organization. "Each comprehensive care clinic does HIV testing, counseling, treatment, and care. The AMPATH Centre in Eldoret has five modules: three for adults located on the ground floor near the entrance, and then a pediatric clinic, 'Module 4,' near the back of the building. There is a pharmacy as well," she said. "It is a one-stop shop." Every county hospital in the MTRH catchment area has at least one CCC, and they all do "differentiated care." Stable HIV clients have groups organized under Population Health that are run by peer leaders. The leader picks up the drugs from a CCC and then distributes them to those in the group every three months, dramatically decreasing travel for most clients.

Rafiki is Module 5 and also has peer leaders, but they are called "peer mentors"—volunteers who work with nearly one thousand clients ages ten to twenty-four. But because the Rafiki Centre's clients are youths, things work a bit differently than at any other CCC and Jane coordinates it all.

A Long Drive from the Lake

Mr. Byrum Angote held out his hand to me, and I shook it. Inside the center, Judy had just introduced me to the crowd as a journalism professor writing a book about Rafiki and AMPATH. Byrum wanted me to know his story. Earlier that morning, he had driven his two sons to the center from Vihiga County, which is just north of Lake Victoria and about a two-hour journey. His oldest son, Michael,[1] was born HIV positive and had been on ARVs since infancy. For the first fourteen years of his son's life, Byrum had taken him to the AMPATH clinic in Mbale Town just a few miles from the family home for his drugs and checkups. But shortly after he and his wife told Michael why he went to the clinic so often, Michael stopped going.

Children who have taken ARVs their entire life are often confused and unhappy when, in early adolescence, they realize that other children do not take daily medicines because they do not have HIV. All too often, they stop taking their medication without telling their parents. The population of adolescents and youths infected with HIV in Kenya is now sizable, primarily because of the increased survival of perinatally infected HIV-positive children through the expansion of HIV testing and treatment services in the early 2000s (Koech et al. 2014).

Byrum and his wife realized their son had stopped taking his ARVs about a year earlier. His viral load had gone from a very low 250 to an alarmingly high 1.2 million. Byrum blamed himself for his son's lapse because he traveled so much for work, but even when parents' jobs do not require travel, adolescents will often stop taking their meds because the desire to be like everyone else is so strong. Most middle-class children like Byrum's attend boarding school and live away from their parents except for breaks every three months or so. While the schools now usually make allowances for positive students to discreetly take their drugs as required, the fact that they are not under the eye of their parents makes it easier for them to fall out of compliance. Peer pressure and the desire for peer acceptance are powerful motivators of unhealthy behavior.

The AMPATH solution has been to provide a space where youth aged ten to twenty-four can be with a peer group that includes others who are positive.

Upon learning that his son was in danger, Byrum began making biweekly visits to Eldoret with Michael for treatment at the Rafiki Centre. "I do this so he doesn't feel alone. At Rafiki he feels welcomed." He enrolled Michael so his son could meet with a cohort of positive adolescents. He said the clinicians there are very friendly and that Michael is now motivated to stay on his medications

1. Michael is not his real name. It has been changed to protect his privacy.

because of the interaction he has with other positive boys and girls at the center.

Because of great advances in the prevention of mother-to-child transmission (PMTCT) of the virus over the last fifteen years, and because Byrum's wife is on antiretroviral therapy (ART) and has an undetectable viral load, Michael's younger siblings are HIV negative, like their father. Even so, Michael's younger brother likes coming to Rafiki because the activities are fun and he feels good being with positive peers. He has lived his whole life with a positive brother, and spending time with other positive youth is comforting.

It is impossible to say how many of the adolescents at the Rafiki Fun Day were positive and how many were negative. The majority no doubt visit the center to collect their drugs and have their viral loads monitored, but many HIV-negative children come to spend time with their siblings or friends in an environment that is supportive and loving. "They feel like they belong and are happy," said Byrum. "I am glad I can bring them here."

Psychological Counseling

Many parents have difficulty dealing with the guilt and stigma that attach to the parents of positive children. Ms. Joyce Oboi is a psychological counselor at the MTRH assigned to the Rafiki Centre. She previously worked on gender-based violence and rape cases and was intrigued by the center's approach to youth, particularly those who were born positive. I asked her about the dynamic between positive adolescents and their parents.

"Usually at the start, the relationship is not quite well because the mother is in denial and the child is in denial, so both of them cannot agree," she said. "Children ask, 'What is this that my parents did that made my siblings not to be positive that they refused to do it to me?' and the mother does not have the language to calm the child or to give the child a true explanation of what happened. Additionally, because of the anger and the stigma and the denial, the mother may throw hurtful words to the child, like, 'If you don't want to take your drugs, you can just as well die, just like your father. It's up to you,'" she said. "Then the child becomes rebellious and says, 'If that is the case, I am not ready to take the drugs and I am ready to die.' Tension in the house can be very high after the child learns his or her status."

"When such kind of clients come to us, we normally try as much as we can to bring the mother on board to help both understand what is going on," she said. "We usually find that disclosure was not done well. Too often the mother was living in denial with a lot of bitterness over how she acquired the virus and so is not willing to help the child understand how she got it," she said. "We sit with mother and child and help them see the denial and see that there is a future." Parents frequently know how to treat their child medically but do not know how to manage the psychological effects.

Even parents who are comfortable with their own status can run into problems with children who are positive because the parents harbor guilt, according to Joyce. "For example, if there are three in the family and they are in high school, the one who is positive may be given a lot of money, a lot of care. These children learn how to manipulate their parents because it's like, 'You are the one who gave me this, so I am your burden and I have to be given more than others.' So many a time you realize that, *eeeeh*, the child says, 'If you don't buy for me this, I will not take the drug,'" Joyce explained. "But as they come to us as counselors, we help them to understand that these children have to grow like any other child, they have to be treated just like any other child. And the children, we help them to understand they are not special; they are just like other children, and they should be able to accept the way their parents are treating them."

A more ideal situation is when the counseling staff are able to advise parents before they disclose their child's status to them. She told me of a session with two positive parents:

> I first ask them how they are taking it. I asked, "How has it been with you?" and the father said, "As the man of the house, I have accepted to live positively, but the problem is, how do we now tell this girl?" So, one of the doctors and I agreed that I would prepare the girl by first talking about diseases that we go through and how we can manage diseases at the MTRH. I asked which of these diseases she feared most, and the girl said "HIV." I asked her why she feared HIV so much, and she said, "When I have it, I might die or people will just know that I did something wrong like involving myself in sexual activities."

Joyce asked the girl to recall what she had been taught in primary school about HIV:

> She knew everything: that transmission can come from sharp objects, through blood transfusion, and from sex, but she was not seeing herself being HIV positive. I asked her to compare between HIV and cancer. "Which one do you fear most?" and she said, "*Yaah*, I hear that when you take the HIV drugs you can live fine, but with the cancer, there is no hope for you." So we dwelled on the negatives and the positives of HIV and later I asked, "Now that we have talked about how if you take your drugs, you live like any other person, you can grow and do everything you have ever wanted to do, could you accept it if your friend were positive?"

The next day, the mother joined the session, and Joyce asked her to share with her daughter how she herself got HIV. "It was very tough for the girl. She wanted to cry,

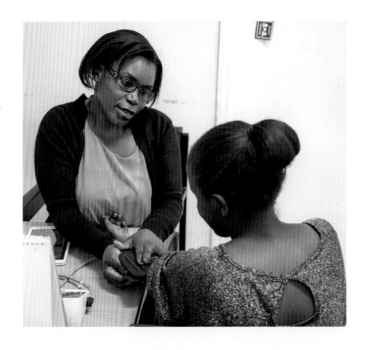

Dolly Nyang'wera, a clinical assistant, does triage during the second week of school break in April. She measured the client's weight, height, blood pressure, and pulse. Changes can indicate problems ranging from poor nutrition to mental health issues.

and she wanted to shout on the mother," Joyce recalled, then continued,

> She was a very brown girl, very beautiful, and we didn't at first know how much we were going to tell her. Then the *daktari* [doctor] stood, talked to her, told her that like her mother, she had been living positively with HIV for the last fourteen years. He told her, "You are still strong, you are still beautiful, there is nothing that has changed. If you continue taking your drugs, you will just live a normal life." By the time she was leaving, she was feeling better and coming to the acceptance. Since then, I have followed the girl up. She is able to talk to the mother and is coming to terms with it all because the disclosure was done rightly . . . and because she has been having the support of the peer counselors here at Rafiki.

The Daktari in Charge

Dr. Edith Apondi Ogalo is the consulting pediatrician at Rafiki Centre. As such, she oversees the entire operation,

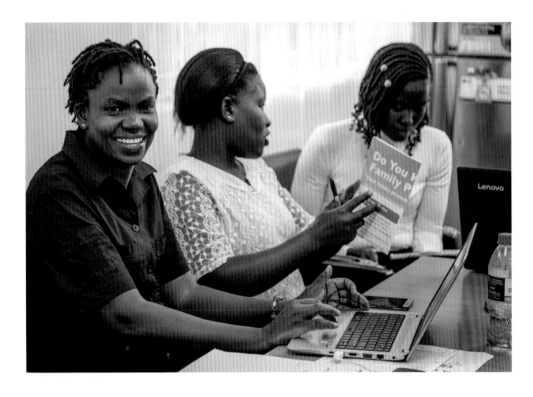

Edith Apondi was the consulting pediatrician at the Rafiki Centre and was instrumental in its establishment in 2016.

although she is quick to say that everyone contributes to its success. She started working for AMPATH in 2004 and has watched the CCCs evolve as treatment of HIV has advanced. ART had proved highly effective and the MoH and AMPATH were growing the number of facilities that could provide the therapy—in high-prevalence areas at first and then in every county in the MTRH's catchment area.

"Because the Ministry of Health was not robust in HIV care early on, those patients were seen separately from the general patients," Apondi recalled. "In that way, HIV became almost a parallel system. With time, we realized drugs were not enough; you needed to provide nutrition, social work, counseling, peer support, and such. We then set up comprehensive care clinics to be comprehensive in the treatment of HIV."

As a pediatrician, she was caring for many children who had been born positive, and she was watching them

grow into youths who were unaware of their illness. By 2010, it was clear that treating older children at adult CCCs was problematic. "Staff at the adult clinics did not have the skills required to handle them. Some of the positive youth would become defiant and become lost to the program. There was an obvious need for something focused on the adolescents," she said.

There were some political challenges to starting an adolescent clinic, however, including issues of space, staff, and supplies. Apondi was tasked with ensuring that the clinic came to be.

"I had a nice team that included Dr. Catherine McDonald from Indiana, Drs. Winstone Nyandiko and Samwel Ayaya from Moi University, and Dr. Paula Braitstein from the University of Toronto. We sat down and negotiated with the hospital and with AMPATH, and we got space which was quickly taken back. We got another space that was demolished to build Shoe4Africa," she recalled. "But eventually we got the wonderful space we have today. The hospital was very kind and provided most of the staff."

The Rafiki Centre is housed in a modest one-story building on the edge of the MTRH campus, surrounded by tall pine trees just about one hundred yards from the Sosiani River. Built a dozen years earlier to store and distribute food to AMPATH clients who needed better nutrition in order for their ARVs to work effectively, it had been empty since that program had been replaced with other FPI initiatives.

The Rafiki Centre "was a departure from the other AMPATH CCCs in that it is staffed by MTRH and run through the Division of Child Health and Paediatrics with substantial AMPATH support under USAID funding," Apondi said, highlighting the fact that the US donor money is restricted to HIV care. "We persuaded the hospital that this new clinic was not just a HIV clinic but was instead 'integrative,'" which means "we have both

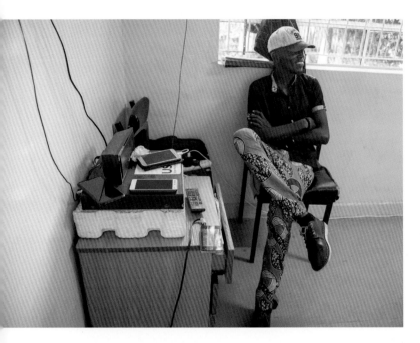

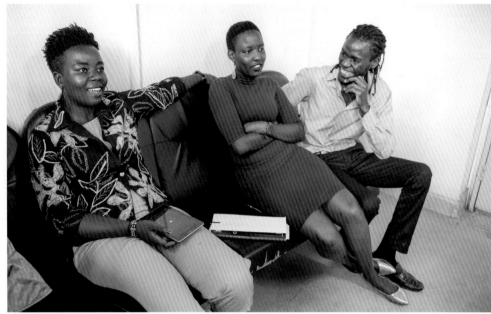

Above left, The dance floor is small, so dancers take turns waiting. Salsa attracts both clients and their friends to the center.

Above right, Joseph Binayo is the salsa dance leader. "Dance is a medicine of its own. It plays a big role in health," he said.

Right, Salsa meets at around five most evenings in the social activities room at the Rafiki Centre. The room is small but plenty big enough for dancing.

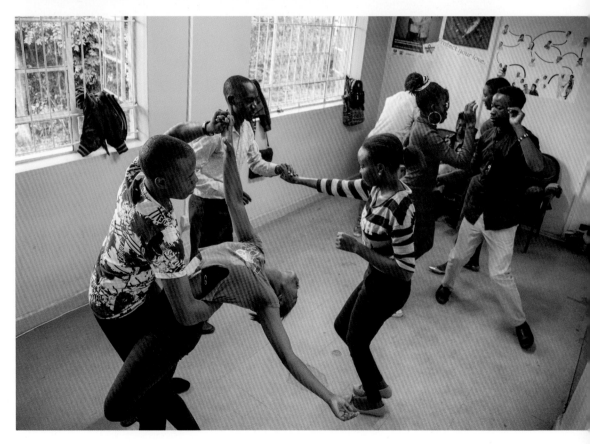

positive and negative clients and we care for all manner of illnesses." Nearly all the staff at Rafiki are MTRH employees, but they receive evaluation, training, and financial support from AMPATH as well as technical support from Moi University and the MTRH directorates of Reproductive Health and of Mental Health & Rehabilitative Services.

Apondi is again quick to point to the real drivers of the change. "It was not like it was our own initiative. The adolescents were pushing us. They were vocal, and they demanded a space. They knew their rights. Today they have taken that space, and they own it," she said with obvious pride.

The Salsa Team

The music being played as Fun Day started may not have been familiar to me, but it didn't surprise me either. A generation ago, Western music, even American country music, was typical on the radios, in *matatus*, and on the streets wherever youth gathered. But as I began bringing IU journalism students to Eldoret, I was increasingly made aware of how African music has come to dominate the airwaves. Youth listen to bonga flava from Tanzania but also Zanzibaran taarab, Swahili and Congolese pop, soukous, zouk, and lots of hip hop, reggae, soul, funk, and rock 'n' roll performed by Africans singing in English, Swahili, and Sheng slang. My IU students were thrilled by the variety and over the last decade have taken home hundreds and hundreds of songs after every visit.

I was surprised by the salsa dancing, however. Salsa was primarily developed by Dominicans and Puerto Ricans living in New York in the late 1960s and early 1970s. Now it is popular across East Africa.

Twenty-four-year-old Mr. Joseph Binayo was the salsa team leader for Rafiki Centre. He started coming to the center in the summer of 2017 because he loves the dance and loves to teach others. He explained to me how integral the Latin dance style is to the social network that makes the center more than just a clinic.

"We come together to dance, to have fun, to live free," he said. "The salsa team's role is to bring people together—boys and girls. It's more than just dancing, it's salsa dancing." He explained that salsa dancing could be done at the clubs in Eldoret as well as at Rafiki but that it is generally associated with sex at the clubs. At Rafiki, however, it helps "remove the idea that boys and girls touching is only about sex," a lesson that is reinforced in the group counseling sessions. "We can come to know each other as people, people who like to dance. We can express ourselves to each other, and even the doctors and nurses here at the center like to dance."

He continued, "We come to Rafiki. We all get information about sexual relations and heathy lifestyles, and some of us get drugs to treat HIV. Mr. Shume explains the drugs to all of us, not just the ones who are HIV positive. That way, we all understand each other better, and at the end of the day, we cannot be against anyone."

"Dance is a medicine of its own. It plays a big role in health," he concluded, and then he invited me to join them that Tuesday afternoon. "Everyone feels welcome to dance at Rafiki."

Nyareso

Counseling sessions, either private with one of the psychologists like Joyce or in groups of clients led by peers, are integral to Rafiki's approach. Navigating adolescence and young adulthood is complicated enough. Doing so with HIV in the household—whether your own, your sibling's, your friend's, or your parent's—compounds the challenge immeasurably. Drugs may keep the virus at bay, but no one is truly healthy until they understand themselves.

Most cases require some sort of social work. Clients often show high levels of depression and schizophrenia, so counselors work closely with psychiatrists at the hospital. Ms. Nyareso Mokaya did her clinical counseling training in the UK and is one of so many who might have stayed abroad had it not been for the rewarding work being done at AMPATH. She said social relationships, romantic

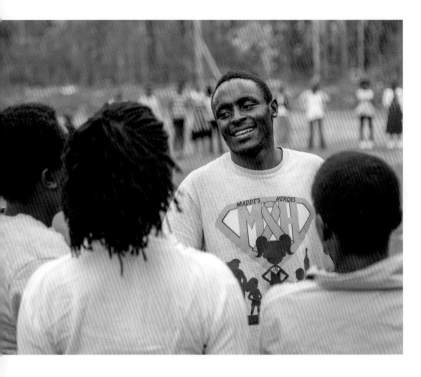

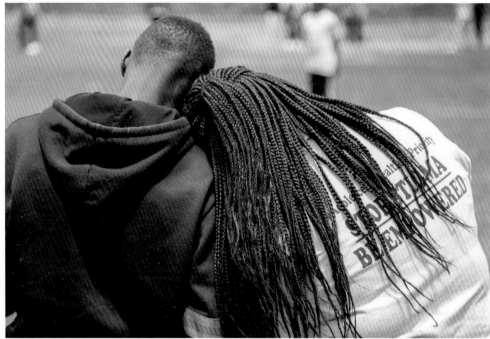

Above left, Hillary Kiptoo is a peer mentor and also an AMPATH client since he was a child.

Above right, Nyareso Mokaya, a social worker, shares a moment with one of the clients. Her shirt says, "Stop Stigma: Be Empowered."

Right, Jane Chemon, Rafiki Centre director, has worked for the MTRH since 2004 and for AMPATH since 2007.

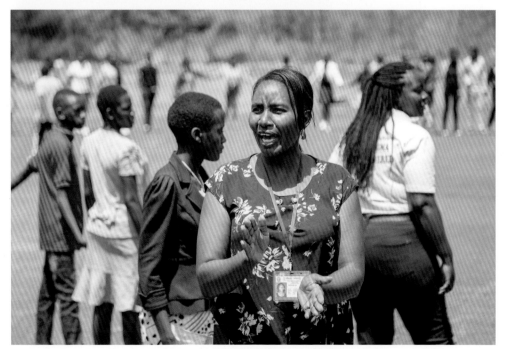

relationships, and other adolescent issues are the bulk of what they deal with. "Group sessions are most useful because the clients get immediate feedback confirming that they are not alone or odd," she said, and then she explained that psychological support groups are used to encourage learning and reflection. "Our goal is that every client meets with a group at least once per year." The groups are homogenous as to key considerations: age, level of vulnerability, and status of treatment. Groups

Top left, Wearing her Leading with Care shirt, Rahab Cheruiyot, a nurse working at Rafiki Centre, joins in the group circle.

Top right, Joel Chanda, a peer mentor, shows a group of young men how to apply a condom in the dark by blindfolding himself with his sweater.

Below, Jane brings one youth into the giant circle formed by peers on the MTRH graduation grounds.

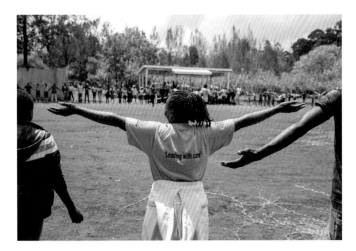

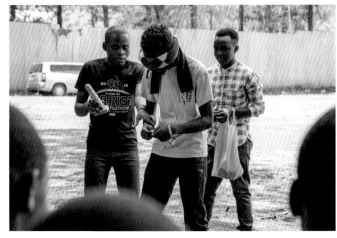

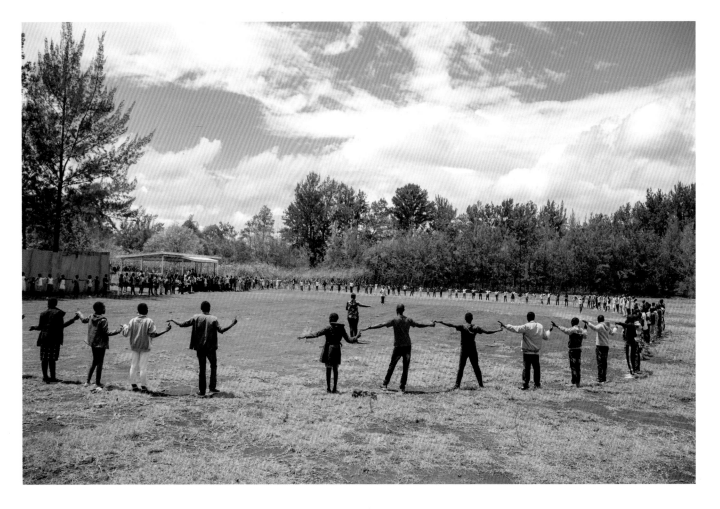

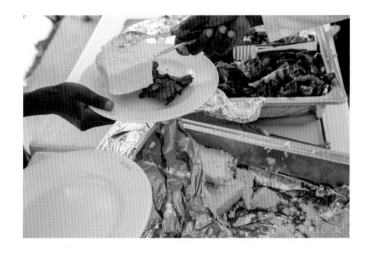

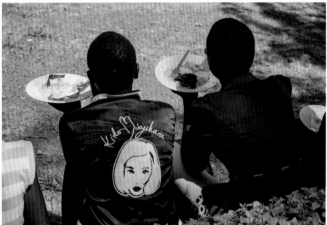

Left and right, Ugali is served with fried chicken and African greens for lunch, which participants eat in the garden in front of the center.

Below, Archie Shume is a clinician and is known for wearing fashionable clothing and making an effort to relate to the youth who visit the center.

meet one to three times per week and more often during the school holidays: April to August. While school is in session, most groups meet Fridays because it is easiest to get away from campus then.

Nyareso offered to ask one of the peer mentors if I could observe a group session but warned me that my attendance would depend on the members. All would have to agree.

Peer Mentors

Mr. Hillary Kiptoo is a peer mentor at Rafiki. Peer interaction is the primary method of engagement, and dozens of people facilitate it. He said he had benefitted from twenty years of AMPATH counseling himself and was proud to now share what he had learned. "The counseling and mentoring I have received caused me to realize that I could live life positively. And I realized I have the skills to help others make the same realization," he said.

When I met with him, he had been through additional training at Rafiki Centre so he could lead group sessions where clients could express their fears and concerns to others. I got to attend part of a session hosted by Hillary and fellow peer counselor Mr. Gideon Kemboi. They met

with six boys and two girls in the same room that later in the day would be filled with salsa dancers. They had all agreed to let the *mzungu* professor into their private space to make photos, but it quickly became clear to me that my presence was dampening the conversation down to pleasantries, despite the fact that Hillary and Gideon had asked probing questions. After making a few photos of the counselors, I thanked them all for allowing me to visit and told them I thought they were lucky to have Rafiki and Hillary and Gideon but that I did not want to spoil their meeting. Smiles came quickly to their faces. They thanked me for coming, but it was pretty clear they were really thanking me for leaving. They needed their privacy.

After the session, Hillary said to me, "Fanya mema kwa wengine na mema atakukujia. Do good to others and good will come to you." He was teaching me a lesson. He said that what I had done by leaving them to their conversations was good for the group. They could see I cared about them.

"You just tell the clients, 'The moment you love yourself is the moment you are headed towards a healthy life.'" He made it sound simple. All people have to do is come to the realization that they are worthy of life, that the virus is something they can live with, and that there is a future. This is a difficult realization for a teenager to make, but peer mentors like Hillary help clients at Rafiki heal and love themselves.

Cool Springs Restaurant

One of my final meetings before leaving Eldoret for Indiana was at Cool Springs Restaurant, just next door to the center, with three peer mentors: Ms. Susan Rono, Mr. Joel Chanda, and Hillary. Like so many of the places AMPATH has touched, the restaurant was started by the FPI about ten years ago to provide employment to clients and on-campus meals to the MTRH staff. We sat under a banda drinking fresh juices and soft drinks. By this point I understood that peer support was the key feature of the center. Healthcare was included, but the clients and others were there because they wanted to be with their friends. Peer mentors were unusually the first friendships they made.

Hillary had been coming to the AMPATH Centre since he was a child. He became a peer mentor as soon as Rafiki opened. Susan had also been one of the first mentors, whereas Joel had just recently joined the peer mentor team. The peer mentors are trained in the basics of counseling, communication skills, HIV, reproductive health, resilience building, and disclosure approaches. They are then entrusted with helping adolescents navigate the hospital setting, leading group counseling sessions, tracing youth who miss their clinic appointments, identifying issues individual youth are facing that interfere with the taking of medication, and general advocacy for the rights of youth in the clinic and the larger hospital. All three of them were excited to explain how Rafiki worked and what it meant to them. I asked Susan what mentors do.

"With every new client, we first introduce them to staff and then show them all around Rafiki Centre so he or she is comfortable," Susan said. "Rafiki deals with a lot. HIV care, reproductive health, cancer screening, counseling psychology, tuberculosis screening, and all that. Everything they do in the CCC modules in the AMPATH Centre, we do here."

Joel jumped in to elaborate. "Before Rafiki there was AMPATH. Children would go to clinic for checkups. They did not know their status. I was in that status. You go to clinic, but you don't know what's the reason you are taking drugs for," he said. "The guys who come to Rafiki, they know. They are fully disclosed. They know, but they may not understand."

Then Hillary chimed in to explain further. "OK, basically, Rafiki is for all youths, not just those that are under care for HIV. Many come when their status is revealed to them in Module 4, but others they come suspecting that they might have been exposed to HIV. They expect to be tested for HIV, but after consulting with the doctor, they usually get a comprehensive screening for many things," he said. "If the person is HIV negative, they can still come here to be with other youths."

Each of them was clearly keen to hear what the others were saying. They nodded in agreement, smiled, and listened. Their mutual respect and fondness were endearing.

Susan continued, "The reason for the youth clinic was to remove the stigma that comes when you enter the AMPATH Centre. When you go there, people suspect your status. But people just don't see you coming into Rafiki," she said, and she waved her hand around as if to reveal the wooded area as distinct from the rest of the hospital campus. "Accepting your status is hard. We told Prof Kimaiyo, 'We need somewhere for privacy.' He said he understood and gave us a building that had previously been for food storage. There was no stigma here. People can come freely. When people ask you, 'Where are you going?' you just say, 'I am going to the youth center. It is just for fun.'"

Joel mentioned that you could enter Rafiki via a parking lot on the edge of the campus, instead of walking through the main hospital grounds. "The thing about Rafiki is that there is no judgment," he said. "I could have dreads and come here and nobody says anything. Youth can come freely, connect with the doctors and then go about their business." He continued, "Before, it was kind of hard coming to AMPATH. I knew my status clear back in primary school. I used to tell people I am going to AMPATH because my aunt works there and I'm just getting my lunch money. There was the fear that I could bump into a neighbor while waiting for clinic. Now I can just say,

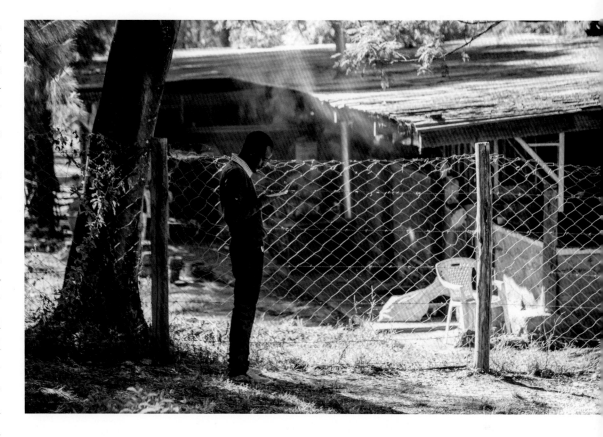

'I'm going to Rafiki,' and they don't think anything about it. Maybe they say they want to come too."

"Basically, Rafiki is a free zone," added Hillary. "It cares for youth, whether it is tuberculosis, HPV, malaria, even PrEP [pre-exposure prophylaxis]. It's not like in the old days where if you were found at AMPATH by your neighbor, you must be positive. Now, if your classmate asks, you can just say, 'I'm coming for malaria,' or if it's a girl, she can say, 'I'm coming for PEP [postexposure prophylaxis].'"

All three said they regularly ask their classmates to come to Rafiki for healthcare, especially sexual healthcare. Hillary said, "Because once a friend comes, they then help others understand Rafiki too. They see that it is here to support youths on all manner of health."

Cool Stream Restaurant is just on the other side of a fence from the Rafiki Centre. Dennis Munyoro, a peer counselor, checks his phone while he waits for some breakfast cooked over an open fire on a chilly morning in January.

Right, Condoms are always free at Rafiki because sexual health is such an essential component of youth health. These sat on the corner of the reception desk just inside the main door.

Facing, Monthly staff meetings are held in the nurses' station at the back of the building. Apondi leads these meetings, but all staff members attend and contribute, whether they are counselors with degrees or peer mentors just out of high school. At this meeting in May 2019, the staff was reviewing records of positive patients with high viral loads. There were seventeen people in a ten-by-ten-foot room, and they reviewed nine patients in less than sixty minutes.

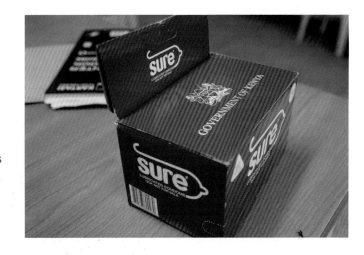

While Rafiki was started to benefit youth who had been born positive, youth too often contract HIV from sexual encounters of their own. HIV infections among fifteen-to-twenty-four-year-olds accounted for a third of all new infections in Kenya in 2017, with young women facing more than double the risk of acquisition compared to their male peers. There are nearly 185,000 youths living with HIV in Kenya, or about two of every one hundred youths (National AIDS Control Council 2018). Sexually transmitted infections (STIs) and unwanted pregnancy are also common health problems.

I had first met Hillary at the group counseling session I briefly attended months earlier, so I asked him about why the sessions are important.

"We all have problems. Maybe someone has not yet accepted the way she is. Maybe she is positive and at session she finds someone who has overcome that problem. The moment they share how they overcame the problem, the person understands they are not alone," he said.

Joel explained that he grew up in his grandmother's home. "When I came to know my status, I asked myself, 'Why me?' I don't know how I got the virus really. I suspect I was born with it, but I don't know because my mom passed away eight years ago. Coming to Rafiki, I've come

to know that I'm not alone. Everyone tells their story, and you hear your own story in their words. It kinda makes you feel comfortable with who you are and who the others are too."

Getting others to share begins with the mentors sharing of themselves, but doing so properly requires training that leads to three key understandings: understand the role, understand the goal, and understand the client. The goal is also three parts: zero missed pills, zero missed appointments, zero viral load. That's Operation Triple Zero. It sounds simple, but it requires a lot of understanding.

They talked about being trained as peer mentors. "We could ask any crazy question about anything, even if it was sexual," Joel said. "There was no discrimination. It wasn't like school where you are not really free to talk." I asked them about sex education in school, knowing that it was legally mandated in Kenya. They all smiled and said it really wasn't useful because it comes when you are too young.

Susan said, "If you are not free with a youth, he or she will not talk with you." She talked about a barrier between kids and their parents when it comes to talking about sexuality. Joel and Hillary nodded as Susan acknowledged that their parents had grown up during a time of civil unrest and that when the AIDS crisis arrived, it made them closed to their children's concerns. "But at Rafiki, you can talk to adults freely," she said.

Peer mentors provide an example to those who come to Rafiki. They are healthy, well adjusted, and positive in their outlook. Susan said,

Before I ask my client anything, I tell my history. I tell my past. I tell them I have been on medication for thirteen years and I cannot give up now. Why should I? I have been LDL [low detectable level of the virus] for thirteen years. It is not easy being LDL, you know, because sometimes you quarrel with your relatives, they discriminate you. I

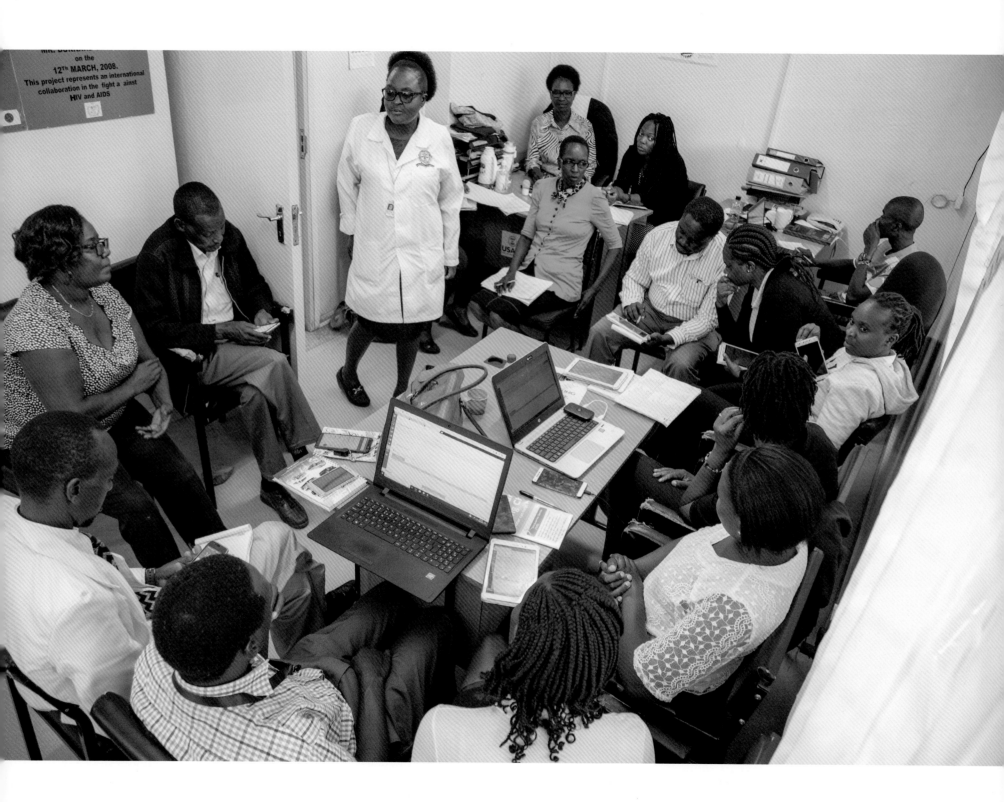

A youth enters the Rafiki Centre on a typical day in January 2019. The center cost more than KSh 4 million to establish and represents a significant investment in adolescent healthcare. It is a joint venture of MTRH, the Moi University School of Medicine, Indiana University, and the county government of Uasin Gishu. The center is the only one of its kind in the region and caters to more than 1,400 youth, including street children, orphans, and vulnerable children.

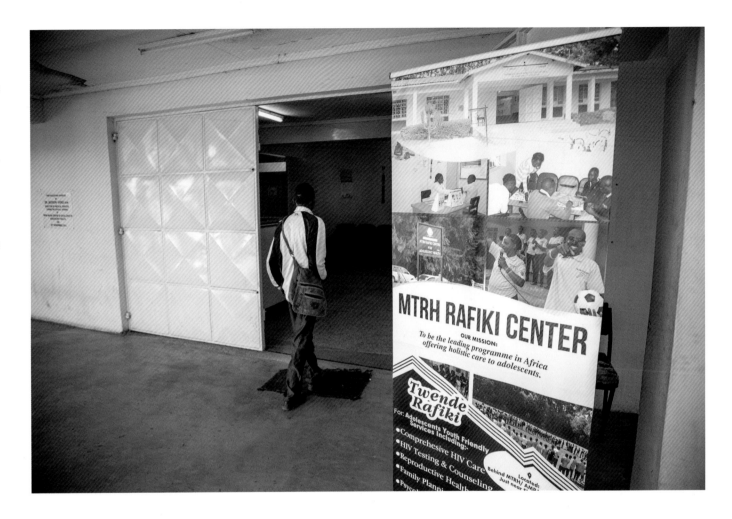

was actually discriminated by my grandmother, but I have to move on. It's my life. Sharing my story with a client will make them open up. Maybe he or she will think, "If you are LDL, why not me?" Being positive is not the end of life.

"Like Susie, I always disclose my status to make them feel free," said Hillary. "I tell them, 'I'm like you.' I've been taking the medication for sixteen years. I am here. HIV is something to be controlled. It is upon me to control it, not it to control me. I must love myself first."

Joel said that "in Africa there are many misconceptions about HIV. But now, anyone can check the fact sheet and know what is what." They told me about the mobile phone app the mentors had created recently. Like

anywhere else in the world, youth in Kenya live with a smartphone in their hand. "The app explains everything," Susan said and gave "U = U" for "Undetectable equals Untransmittable" as an example. "It is code for 'if you are undetectable, you cannot transmit the virus to your partner during sex.' HIV does not mean you cannot have a partner. We are saying, 'If you love them, take care of them.'" The app also explains that even when you are undetectable and therefore unable to transmit HIV, you must still use protection because the risk of pregnancy and STDs remains. The mentors said there are always condoms freely distributed at Rafiki because condoms protect against so many problems.

Susan continued, "It's just like any other disease." Immediately Joel said, "You can lead a normal life," and Susan responded, "like any other person," and then in unison, Hillary and Susan said the same thing: "So long as you take your drugs, everything is OK."

Hillary said, "You see, everybody at Rafiki is friendly—the nurses, the doctors, the counselors. What the youths do, the doctors do. You can find a doctor running, dancing, enjoying. Doctors at the MTRH might find it weird to dance. Personally, I can tell the doctors here anything, anything." Joel then added, "There is that kind of connection they have with us, the peer mentors and everyone who comes."

Joel said, "It takes time for new clients to know that everyone here can be trusted." Hillary added, "Sometimes the doctor knows more about the child than the parents,"

and then when I said, "and you guys know more too," they laughed and agreed that they do.

Susan said, "Jane knows us more because she has been with us since we were children," and Joel continued, "She is like a mother to us." Susan then added, "Personally, I never knew my mom, so I call Jane *mama kwa wote*," which means mother to all. "For me, Rafiki is home," concluded Susan, and the others nodded in agreement.

Hillary expressed hope that other hospitals in Kenya will create their own Rafiki Centres. He said, "The moment you have someplace just for the youths, you can build home."

I ask them to tell me the most important thing about Rafiki Centre. Joel replied, "Prof, if someone comes to you and says, 'What is Rafiki?' you can just tell them Rafiki is home. It's just home."

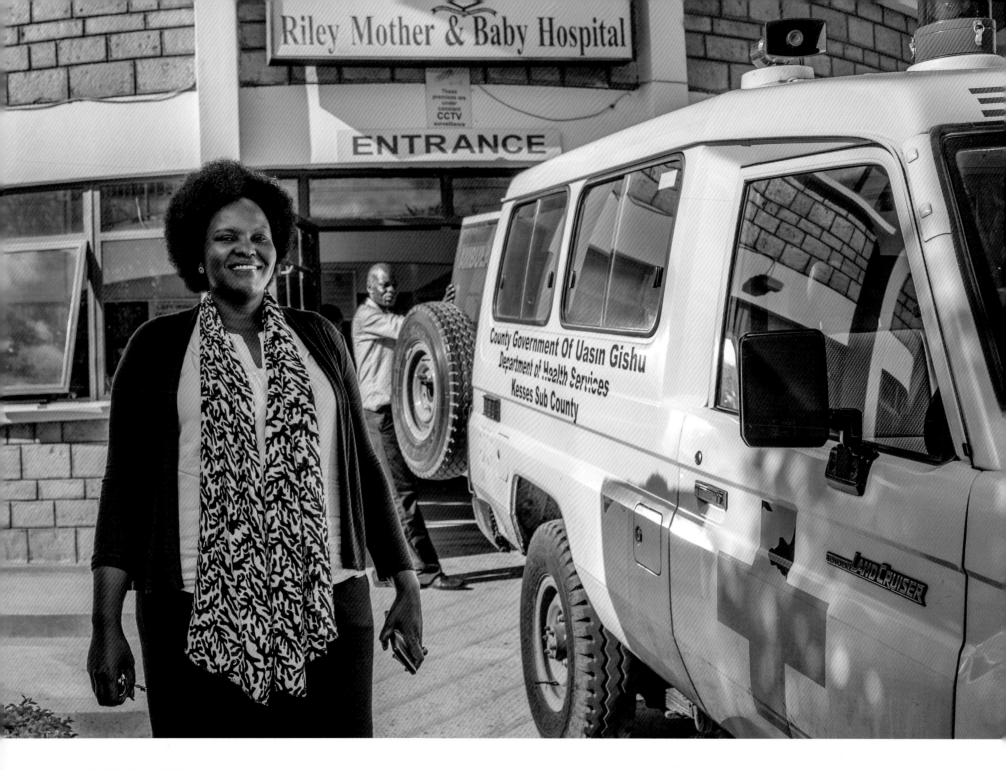

Dr. Julia Songok thinks of herself as a "child of AMPATH," having been a medical student of doctors like Haroun Mengech, James Lemons, and others who are now her medical colleagues in Kenya and North America.

PART THREE

LEADERSHIP PROFILES

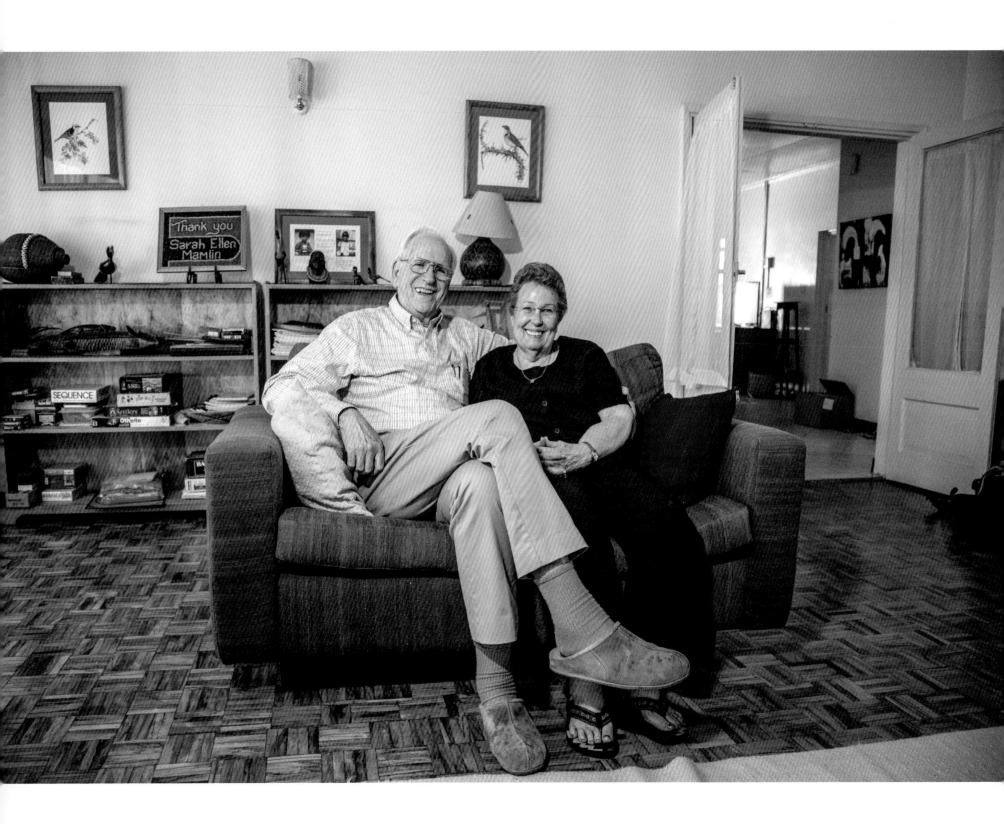

CHAPTER EIGHT

The Leadership

Joe Mamlin

For nearly thirteen years, Joe and Sarah Ellen Mamlin lived in a home surrounded by bougainvillea, a hearty vine that climbs over fences and walls and blooms year-round in red, pink, and magenta. The house is just across the lane from the IU House, a complex of eight buildings where short-term residents visiting AMPATH stay and where the Mamlins lived when they started their retirement visit in 2000.

Joe and I sat in a small banda, a thatched, round-roofed, open-walled hut with a table and four chairs nestled in the foliage about fifteen feet from the front door. With wind chimes tinkling from the porch in the ever-present gentle breeze, Joe immediately established the ground rules for the interview. This was not to be a book about Joe Mamlin. He stated, "I have almost no interest in that. I wouldn't be a very active participant in a book about me." It was as I expected. In a land where elders are afforded great respect and leaders are often credited with successes beyond their actual accomplishments, Joe eschews such adoration. He is a humble man who takes pride in the success of colleagues and claims little for himself.

I started our conversation by asking him to reflect on a prediction he had made in Fran Quigley's 2009 book about AMPATH ten years earlier. Joe had said, "Kenya is preparing to rise to the heights never dreamed of in Africa" (140). That was in 2008. For the first two months of that year, the country had been convulsed by tribal

Facing, For twenty years, Joe and Sarah Ellen Mamlin lived in a four-bedroom house surrounded by gardens in Elgon View Estates, a short walk from the hospital where they spent their working days. The couple raised their Kenyan son, Dino Martins, here and hosted hundreds of guests from Kenya and North America. They usually took their evening meals at the IU House, the boarding house just across the lane, so they could share stories with short-term visitors and other long-term residents around the communal tables there. Joe was one of the founding members of AMPATH and former director of Wishard Memorial Hospital in Indianapolis.

violence following a botched election. In the Great Rift Valley, hundreds of mainly Kikuyu people had been killed and maimed in machete attacks by gangs of Kalenjin people. The largest single loss of life happened just miles from Eldoret when a church providing shelter from the violence for two hundred people was set on fire by rioters, killing thirty-five. Most of the wounded were taken to the MTRH, where Joe and other IU doctors treated them. Fran recalled Joe having said, "This will go down as the worst day of my life. . . . In the emergency room, I step over the dead to reach for those dying" (135).

For two months, IU House provided refuge to more than 130 people as the violence against the Kikuyus raged. Most were medical workers and their families assigned to the MTRH by the Ministry of Health and therefore living outside their traditional tribal homelands. After weeks of negotiation while violence racked the country, a peace agreement brokered by former UN secretary general Kofi Annan was reached on February 28. Joe had lived as close to this terrible violence as any foreigner in the country. At the time, his prediction of a bright future sounded counterintuitive. Kenya seemed to be coming apart, not moving forward. But he saw more clearly than most international commentators how determined Kenyans were to build a bright future. Now, ten years later and just a few days before he and Sarah Ellen would move back home to Indiana, Joe wanted to talk about where AMPATH had been and where it was going.

"I think it's gone in a positive direction. We haven't seen that return of violence that we had. That's one thing. There's more talk at least of tackling one of the great diseases in Kenya—corruption," he said, calling out the root cause of that postelection violence and praising that "very noble goals have been put out by the current administration." He continued, "One is, of course . . . close to our hearts is a commitment by 2020 to have universal health insurance"—and, with that, affordable universal healthcare for every Kenyan. He pointed to the effects of the new constitution passed in 2010 as empowering local leaders and giving them the resources to achieve universal healthcare in a country with a healthcare system still struggling to end the HIV/AIDS epidemic.

Joe remains ever optimistic. His understanding of future possibilities is grounded in a thoughtful appreciation and critical analysis of the history of the partnership between two medical schools in Indiana and Eldoret that he helped start three decades earlier. He described it as composed of three epochs.

The first epoch was marked by collaborative efforts to build medical capacity. Joe, Bob Einterz, and others from IU had joined with Haroun Mengech thirty years earlier as he and the government's Ministry of Health established the country's second medical school. The president at the time, Daniel arap Moi, announced the goal just before Joe and Bob's first visit in 1988. They were impressed with Mengech's innovative ideas about pedagogy and decided they could work with him and the leadership team he gathered out on the western edge of the country.

Joe credited those Kenyan visionaries as leading the collaboration that marked that first epoch. "North Americans were certainly putting their shoulder to the task under Kenyan leadership to move toward a school that is recognized now as a fine school. It was the Kenyan leadership that attracted us here in the first place," he stated. In this beginning, the idea of leading with care first came to the fore. Throughout the early years,

the school stayed faithful to its mission of being sensitive to the community in which it lived and that it served. It's always placed its students out in rural health centers as part of their training. It's sustained an aura of being responsive to the population it serves and not just the self-interest of its doctors. . . . I think of the first ten years as just being a part of a med school getting its bearings and recognition. I think that was wonderful. But it's foundational for what was the next step [the partnership's response to the HIV/AIDS epidemic at the start of the project's second decade]. All that was due to the wisdom of Indiana University that sent a ragtag team out looking for a place to do mischief in 1988.

The foundation built during the first epoch was solid. A response to AIDS could be built upon it.

"No one then ever discussed confronting a pandemic called HIV as we were talking about engaging with med school, nor did anyone raise his hand and say, 'I think this is in the epicenter of the world's greatest pandemic.' I don't believe that conversation occurred," he recalled. But the IU-Kenya Partnership did step up and worked alongside Kenyans to recast HIV from a death sentence into a chronic condition. Joe stated, "I would say the last twenty years has been proving the wisdom of that founding philosophy. We have been showing the ability of an academic medical center to respond to the real hurt of the society in which it was growing. The partnership built credibility, and it empowered Kenyans to drive this thing forward from HIV crisis to universal healthcare."

Joe talked of how the years of collaboration had forged a bond between the folks at the medical school and the hospital system that could take on any challenge. "For this collaboration to dare to knock on the door the Ministry of Health and say, 'Your mess is our mess. How can we join hands here and take this on as a team?' Well, that's really what AMPATH is really all about," he said. While neither the acronym it is now known by nor the slogan that symbolizes its approach had been formulated in 2001, the principles that underpinned AMPATH's Leading with Care motto were firmly entrenched in the ethos of the still-young medical school. He stated, "We literally put 'care first' into every step along the way. I think that was a

stretch for Kenya, and it was a stretch for North America, but it was all a natural outgrowth of that first effort" of creating a medical school focused on practical training.

The notable event that likely marks the beginning of this second epoch was Joe's discovery of Daniel Ochieng in a bed in Bay 3 of the MTRH in 2001. Daniel was a Moi medical student—Joe's student. He was quietly dying from AIDS instead of attending classes. Joe was compelled to do something extraordinary and transformed Daniel into the first Kenyan in a public hospital to receive antiretroviral drugs to treat HIV. Virtually no Africans were being treated with the drugs at the time.

Joe contacted Bob Einterz at IU and requested help in treating Daniel. "Joe Wheat, an infectious disease specialist in the Department of Medicine, provided the $1,000 per month required to treat Daniel," Joe said. "And a few months later, Dr. Wheat surprised us all with a donation to cover the treatment of an additional forty patients. That small beginning was followed by key funding from a family foundation in Canada and, ultimately, support from the USAID/PEPFAR initiative," a series of multimillion-dollar grants from USAID supported by PEPFAR.

"If you had looked at that first room with that first patient, you'd have seen a slow addition of one more room over there and then a clinic over there. Today that one room has grown into probably one the largest HIV programs in the world," he said. "AMPATH now provides about 180,000 people with HIV care. That one room is now maybe eight hundred clinics. I think that's a wonderful story."

It is a wonderfully powerful story, not just because of Joe's insistence that he could not stand by as people died but also because of the generous financial support given by folks back in Indiana to assist in the fight. Small foundations and personal donations provided the money used to build necessary infrastructure. Within three years of Ochieng's recovery, AMPATH was receiving US government assistance and thousands of people were being treated. Today it is tens of millions of dollars and tens of thousands of patients. But according to Joe, the key to the current success was outstanding Kenyan leadership. AMPATH had an exemplary reputation for fiscal management and patient care, and that garnered genuine trust from ordinary Kenyans and US officials.

"Show me another place where the US government is awarding $60, $70, $80 million grants . . . to an institution in the developing world," he said. I could not, because AMPATH in Eldoret is the only place where it is happening. While the first two multimillion-dollar grants awarded to AMPATH from USAID went to Indiana University as the primary investigator, subsequent grants starting in 2012 have been awarded directly to the MTRH. A key marker of the success of the IU-Kenya Partnership is the enhanced capacity of Kenyan leadership, which now leads one of the first and largest USAID/PEPFAR grants awarded to a host country.

"That our government gives that much money to Kenyans here speaks to the level of success this Kenyan leadership has achieved," he said. "It's a story about Kenyans leading Americans." Joe is keen on this point. "The leadership that's emerged and their capacity to drive their own future is remarkable." He takes obvious pride in how well the capacity building of the first epoch led to the solutions of the second epoch and has now positioned AMPATH to play a major role in the provision of universal healthcare during the third epoch. Joe continued:

> You know when a plant grows and you kind of watch for a while? It's interesting to see what fruit comes popping out. I think we're beginning to see the most delicious fruit of this effort, this thirty-year journey we've been on. Now it's just at its infancy of engaging in population health. Sure, there was an epidemic within the population, but the real

monster, as I've always said, is three headed. It's got one head called poverty, it's got one head called hunger, and one called disease. And you can't get that monster to lie down until you go after all three of them.

Joe is certain that the population health initiative underway now is the natural outflow of the capacity building of the first epoch and the provision of emergency care during the second. He said, "Population health is just as visionary as was the idea that we could start a med school responsive to the community back in epoch one." He believes Kenyans are prepared to say, "Let's do the whole thing." He commented, "We were talking about this as the next right step before the president of Kenya made his commitment toward universal health coverage. Our initiative just fits like a glove going on a hand. It is the natural thing to do."

Like the wise old professor he has been since his days as chief of medicine at Wishard Memorial Hospital when it was the IU School of Medicine's teaching facility in Indianapolis, Joe explained the lessons today's AMPATH leaders learned while fighting AIDS and how those hard-won lessons have prepared them for the current epoch. "To do HIV care, you had to get out into the villages, and you had to get into everybody's home. We worked door to door to stop that pandemic. It wasn't just something interesting that showed up in your clinic," he recalled.

For Joe, the essential realization was that you had to go to where people lived, oftentimes far beyond the paved road and the dirt road after that. He said, "You didn't do it with doctors. It was not work for doctors. It was work for community workers, social workers, nutritionists, clinical officers, nurses, community health workers, all working in the villages."

Of course, doctors had played a huge role, but Joe's point was that the bulk of patient care was done by staff who had little formal training beyond certificates and diplomas. The infrastructure AMPATH built to combat AIDS was exactly what was needed to provide universal healthcare. Both prevention and treatment of HIV required village-level early intervention before AIDS put people on their deathbed and ideally before HIV was transmitted in the first place.

Universal healthcare "is not just caring for a patient who's had a stroke. You need to find hypertension ten years before the stroke and treat it. It's not just providing good care for a patient with cervical cancer, it's preventing it by screening for cervical cancer out in the village. You must dare to care about mental health and to care about indoor air pollution or water purity or whatever it is that burdens the population," he said.

He points to the leadership of Sylvester Kimaiyo, who is currently the head of AMPATH Plus, the part of AMPATH focused exclusively on HIV/AIDS. Joe commented, "He's under tremendous pressure to deliver HIV results. Everyone's looking down his back, and now we're saying we've got to contaminate every one of those HIV clinics that were built over the last twenty years with hypertension, diabetes, cancer detection, mental health screenings, and we have to get everyone multitasking in all directions. Oh my God!" As his friend Kimaiyo and all the AMPATH leadership admit, foreign donations will never provide enough money to fund Kenya's healthcare needs. Sustainable care for all will have to be paid for by Kenyans. They can do it by expanding the care at AMPATH clinics from HIV to all manner of maladies—and especially prevention.

"The movement toward population health with universal insurance is a byword for doing what common sense tells you ought to be. . . . It's an extremely exciting time," he said, but with a nod to the fact that he will not be among the leadership that will establish a population health system that delivers universal healthcare paid for by fair and affordable national insurance. That is now up to those who follow in Joe's footsteps.

I asked him about his colleagues in the AMPATH Consortium, which then included fifteen North American medical schools working alongside IU. "We're not here just to do medicine," he said. "I would say there are two things that are critically important. One is to be a part of giving birth to a generation of Kenyans who can dream with vision, who can organize their thoughts, create strategic approaches, and realize that they can make it happen. The other one is just as important. Each of us has an opportunity to become better people ourselves."

Joe has done much to achieve that first goal. Nearly every doctor and nurse I talked with in Eldoret told me I needed to write a book about "Prof Mamlin." They admire him for his ability to empower and inspire them. But Joe's second point here is about his fellow Westerners— the *wazungu*, as foreign white folks are known. Joe has witnessed dozens and dozens of young medical students and residents, as well as dozens more senior doctors and pharmacists, experience the transformative power of the academic model he helped put in place thirty years ago. He is just as impressed by the effect AMPATH has had on the *wazungu* as the effect it has had on the Kenyans.

According to Joe, "I think we have found a way of collaborating that may not have been seen before" in North-South partnerships. "It's been good for individual North Americans like myself and perhaps has made me a somewhat better person," he confided. "Having engaged this struggle, I hope the day will come when the people of Indiana will look at it and say, 'Hmm. Strange, painful, odd, unexpected, but by George they got out and did that.'" He credits IU leadership for tolerating the radicalness of their main idea—the notion that personal relationships nourished by patient care had to be grown over the long, long run. "You don't know how grateful I am that they've tolerated that from us. It's a very important characteristic of a great university," he said.

Joe hopes the academic model expands beyond Kenya soon. He pointed to a project at the University of Texas Medical School to partner with a hospital in Mexico and another project AMPATH leadership is helping with in northern Ghana. I asked him if he thought they would succeed. "As long as they stick to the mission statement, 'care leads the way,'" he replied, claiming that the idea behind that simple phrase is radically different from other approaches. "When you say care leads the way, you create a natural laboratory for your research, and, lo and behold, it's more competitive than research done elsewhere. It's the environment for your education. Lo and behold, it's learning that is more relevant. There's a richness that comes from that initial statement, Leading with Care. It embodies the notion of population health because care for the population is *out front* at all times." Leading with Care has been the fundamental lesson of the Moi medical school since the first day. It is monogramed on the aprons and lab coats that nurses, doctors, clinicians, and technicians wear at the MTRH and every clinic in the twelve counties AMPATH serves.

Joe sees the lessons learned in Eldoret as applicable in Indiana as they have been in Kenya. "What we're doing here can be informative to North America, just as what North America is doing is informative here. We need to listen and learn from each other. If we can do something in a Kenyan county called Usain Gishu, we can do the same in an Indiana county called Marion," he said.

I think there are lessons here we can share back and forth. . . . As world citizens, we need to ask, "What are we learning as a world community that can be instructive bidirectionally." I've learned to say to young [medical and pharmacy students] coming here, if you want to do global health, understand it's all about the glasses you wear. It's

the prism through which you look at fellow human beings. It's not geography. If you have to travel to do global health, you miss the point. You can do global health in Muncie. You can do global health in Bloomington. You can do global health in Eldoret.

Lots of people had asked him what he would do with his time back in Indianapolis, and so did I. He responded, "All I've ever done with my time is to struggle mightily to refine my personal values and to make sure my daily activities were in harmony with them. There's no reason why I can't keep doing that."

Sylvester Kimaiyo

Dr. Sylvester Kimaiyo sat in the same corner office where I had first met him in 2009. The open casement windows allowed Eldoret's reliably gentle breeze to animate the sheer white curtains so they seemed to dance in the background. Kimaiyo is a tall man who sits forward in his chair as if he is about to reach across the desk and take your hand. He smiles easily. He speaks with enthusiasm.

Kimaiyo is the executive director of AMPATH Care and chief of party of AMPATH Plus. He is charged with the daily running of AMPATH. He also lectures at Moi University and does rounds in the MTRH. Kimaiyo believes that "part of the job description of any AMPATH physician, regardless of their other roles, is to see patients."

Ten years ago, I was planning to bring journalism students from IU Bloomington to report on AMPATH. I had permission from the North American side from the codirector, Bob Einterz, in Indianapolis, but not from the Kenyan side. I had been in Nairobi training journalists and took a side trip over to Eldoret. I asked Kimaiyo if he would support my course by giving my students access to his staff, and he replied, "Of course, why not?" I felt welcomed then, and I have felt comfortable in his presence ever since.

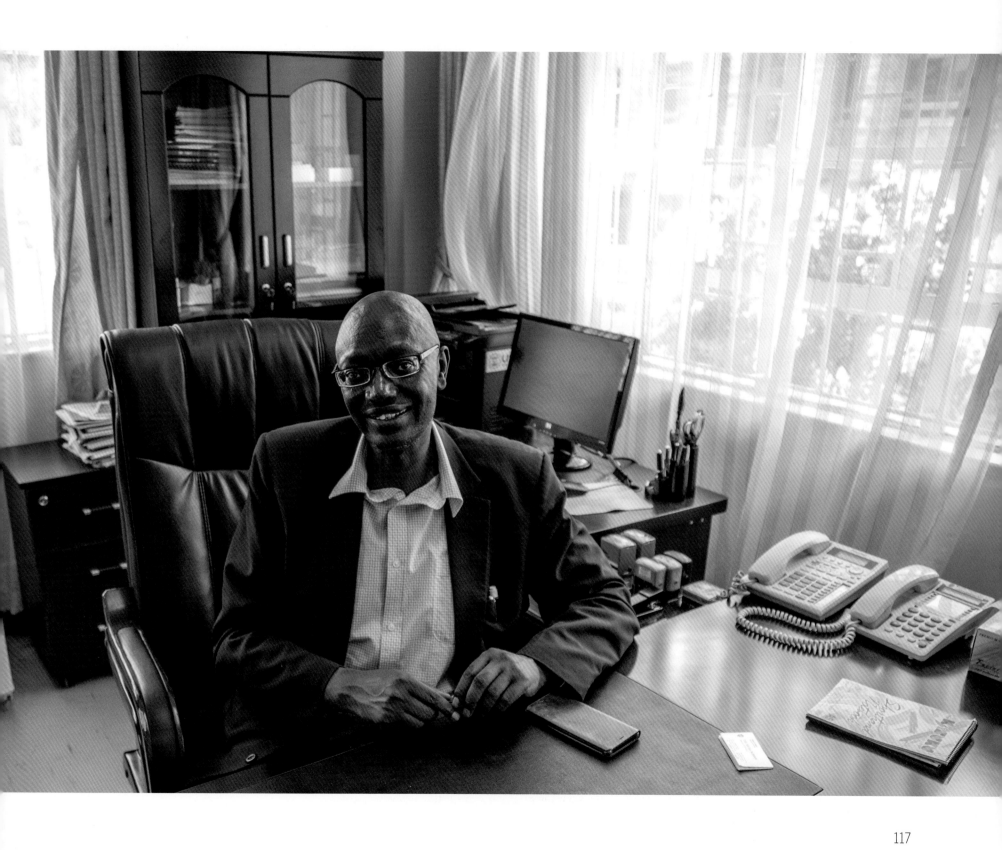

Like all Kenyans he is welcoming in a way that can startle a Westerner. The Swahili word for welcome is *karibu*, and it is always said with an extended hand in anticipation of the gentle handshake that starts virtually every conversation. Unlike most Kenyans, however, Kimaiyo is willing to talk about the toughest issue—money—directly and honestly. As head of AMPATH Plus, the side of the program that oversees programs sponsored primarily by USAID, he manages a lot of money. Tens of millions of dollars from the US are provided each year to address the HIV epidemic, and since 2013, those dollars have been deposited directly into Kenyan hands at MTRH. At the time of our interview in April 2019, signals from Washington suggested the US government might soon decrease funding for HIV/AIDS programs in Africa (Gathura 2019).

I reminded him that it had been six years since I had last talked with him and that at that time, he had been noticeably anxious about the USAID funding. "You know that was a tough, tough period. We had worked with IU from 2001 when we started AMPATH—Bob Einterz and the whole team. Professor Mamlin was here, but the legal custodian for most of the projects was Bob in Indy. We depended a lot on Bob," he recalled. "There were advantages and disadvantages, of course, but it was good that IU had the grant because I was protected."

Since the first PEPFAR award in 2003, Indiana University had been the "prime." As such, IU managed grant administration, including fiscal audits. The arrangement "flipped" in 2012 when USAID awarded $74 million over five years directly to MTRH. Kimaiyo became the man responsible for program implementation and accounting (Einterz 2015). "We had been equal partners for so long. We did not know the difference between AMPATH and MTRH," he said. "Now, suddenly, we had all the responsibilities. USAID would say they don't know IU. They only know their prime, and that was us."

"It was a moment of anxiety, actually. There was excitement, but looking back, and this is interesting, Bob had actually allowed us all along to speak directly to USAID," he said. "Without really knowing, he had all along been training us to take over. . . . We grew up like that."

AMPATH Plus is now the name of the side of the partnership that focuses exclusively on HIV/AIDS. It collaborates with the Population Health team, but its budget is distinct, and it even has its own accounting and management operation. "We have grown bigger. Around 2012, we were probably about 60,000 patients on HIV treatment. Now we are almost 180,000. Yeah. So, things have changed," Kimaiyo said.

I suggested that 2012 was the point at which Kenyans starting taking the lead from what had been a project driven more by IU and the consortium. But Kimaiyo pushed back. He knows the longer history well. "I want to classify that a bit," he said. "From 1990, IU was involved in building and developing the curricula for the upcoming medical school. But it was *our* project. There was no lead, there was only partnership. All those MOUs [memorandums of understanding] and agreements were preparation for what was to come administratively."

In 2000, Kimaiyo was in his fourth year of medical studies at the University of Nairobi. "The new school at Moi had not yet graduated any students. I left to go to Indianapolis for my fellowship training in 2000—the year Mamlin arrived here in Eldoret. While I was at IU for two years, there were a lot of new things to me—the Internet, the email, learning how to use PowerPoint, how to write proposals, how to participate in research. I spent time in cardiology, and I spent time in HIV," he said.

While Kimaiyo was a world away in Indianapolis, at home his professors were creating AMPATH, the organization built to confront the HIV/AIDS epidemic in western Kenya. Kimaiyo was learning skills he would soon contribute to the new operation. "A gentleman called Dr. Joe Wheat was in HIV at IU. He adopted me and said we would do everything together. I still did cardiology, but I spent time in the HIV clinic twice a week," he said. "I saw a lot in that clinic."

"In May 2002 I arrived back in Eldoret, and Joe Mamlin saw me as fully trained in HIV in America. But he had to train me in HIV in Kenya. I had been doing HIV care in the United States where any test you wanted, it was there. Any of the medicines you wanted, it was all there. And when I came back here, I was told, 'These are the three or four medicines that we have,'" he recalled. "When I came back, I think we had money to treat forty patients." But there were thousands of people testing positive for HIV at the time.

He told me about the small grants they received from places like the Purple View Family Foundation that allowed them to increase patient load, but they were still only able to scratch the surface of the epidemic that was killing hundreds every month. "By late 2003, when President Bush announced in the State of the Union address that they were going to create PEPFAR, we were over a thousand patients, almost two thousand patients on treatment. We were big." Kimaiyo remembered Joe saying that "something will happen," and he then exclaimed, "And it did!"

Because AMPATH was already treating far more HIV-positive patients than any other organization in Africa, both the CDC and USAID asked them to make funding applications. Joe asked Kimaiyo which they should choose, and Kimaiyo recalled saying, "USAID is very good, but CDC is very good too. I remember honestly telling him, 'As a Kenyan amid all this desperation—let's take both!'"

They did, and they ended up with enough funding to treat fifteen thousand patients with CDC money and another fifteen thousand with USAID money. They were applying the lessons they had learned from the smaller grants and learning how to work with the two biggest US funding agencies.

Kimaiyo momentarily thought back to the days before his IU fellowship and the big grants from USAID, back to the late 1990s when he was a student on the wards of the MTRH. He said, "Anybody who was diagnosed with HIV also had AIDS because we didn't have easy screening tools. I remember all those patients. You know I had my own sister who died from AIDS in 1997. I had colleagues, like brothers and sisters, who died. There was nothing we could do."

"As I was leaving for Indiana in 2000, I had a panel of fifteen patients I had been following. Joe told me, 'You know what, something will happen.' I told him, 'Joe, here are my fifteen patients, just in case you can get them something,'" he recalled. "When I came back in 2002, most of those patients were still alive because they had been offered treatment. That was really an inspiration going forward."

I asked him why AMPATH has succeeded. He replied, "Well, that's a hard question, but I think, first of all, it has been the philosophy that was put there all along, Leading with Care." As I had come to understand, that motto was not simply that taking care of patients was prioritized over research. "Leading" meant working together to provide care for the entire community.

"We were together in the wards, we were together in the clinics, we were together in the outstations, whether there was funding or not," he said. "We have always had a direction to follow. We wanted to get rid of HIV. We wanted to control HIV. We wanted to prevent HIV. And now we want to prevent cancer. We want to treat cancer. We want to put it under control, and we are doing it fast. It is the continuity of our efforts."

"If you look at the people since 1988, it's a lot of the same people," he said. "It's Bob. It's Joe. It's me. It is a whole community, both on the US side and here. . . . It has been the presence of IU in Eldoret throughout the years. There's always somebody here. We have Adrian [Gardner] and his family now. Bob comes and goes. You have the team that is in surgery, somebody in pharmacy. That's continuity, and they're building trust. What I also see is that it is mutual, you know."

"When I look at the Moi University School of Medicine, almost everybody has been able to do something at Indianapolis or Toronto, or someplace where there's a consortium member," he said. "They come here. We go there."

"And while it's still Leading with Care, now it's also research. At first, my colleagues here were a bit slow in doing research," he continued before explaining that AMPATH has always insisted that Kenyans should earn authorship on academic papers led by consortium members from the West. "Now, people are writing proposals directly to NIH [National Institutes of Health in the US], and they get them," he said. "In 2000, I had zero academic publications. Right now, I have close to one hundred."

If Kimaiyo measures success in patient numbers and research journal articles, he nevertheless recognizes the role money plays in motivating people to do their best. "What we have done also is we . . ." He pauses and then says, "This is tricky. We have provided financial compensation to our consultants."

In Kenya, like Britain, a consultant is a senior hospital-based physician or surgeon who has completed all of his or her specialist training. These consultants are the top of the hierarchy and have great responsibility for patient care. In 1990, Kenya ruled that consultants at government hospitals could do part-time private practice. In this way, the government could keep their pay in line with other

highly paid government workers, but the consultants could earn more money than most government employees by working longer hours. Up to 50 percent of their time could be spent at clinics they themselves owned.

"Some people misuse this," he said. "In Nairobi, for example, you can hardly get the teachers teaching students. They are out in their private practice. So, what we did here is that we bought that time from the consultants. . . . There are some here who don't do any private practice. Instead, they work in AMPATH. Either that they have written a grant or they are in the care program, but they are compensated financially."

"The bad side of that is that the [extra] compensation has made us a little expensive," he admitted. AMPATH buys the consultants' private-practice time using overhead charged to the various organizations that fund AMPATH research. Major research hospitals competing for those research grants, like Makerere University in Uganda or Muhimbili University in Tanzania, submit proposals with lower costs than the MTRH can offer because their doctors are paid only the government wage.

"Sometimes the grants go there instead of here because what we ask is expensive," he said. "But then they come back to AMPATH because we can deliver. It's a tricky balance. But it's a balance game that folks in Uganda and Tanzania and Malawi don't get to play at all. They can't turn down offers."

AMPATH provides advantages other places do not. They have the Research and Sponsored Projects Office (RSPO), a quasi-independent accounting office that ensures that funds are spent properly and to the exacting standards of USAID. They have an extensive electronic data repository built over decades of careful patient data collection and management using the AMPATH Medical Record System, a web-based, open-source medical records system that now holds the largest clinical data repository in Africa. They have the institutional support of the MTRH, Moi University, and the AMPATH Consortium. And then there is the scope of the operation.

"We have very many patients," he said. "If you are looking for the sample size, we've got it. Yeah. We overshoot it. We have the rural, semi-desert in West Pokot. We have urban Eldoret and Kisumu. We have the border area, and we have the lake [Lake Victoria, the world's second largest]. We have a varied area to draw upon in terms of culture, environment, and disease patterns."

Without me asking, Kimaiyo starts telling me about sustainability and the future. He says this is the question the press always asks, and he starts by asking me, "If all the donors go, do you close shop?" He has a ready answer: "And we say no. . . . We may reduce, but we will not stop because it's still the mandate of Moi University and MTRH to treat our patients," he said, and then he went on to talk about the real solution to sustainability. "The population health that you see happening is our future. If we get an insured population, that will take over from all this donor support, if we manage it well. Yeah."

The insurance plan is the National Hospital Insurance Fund. The national government is expanding the NHIF, and AMPATH has projects to encourage people to sign up across the region. For the equivalent of five dollars a month, the entire family gets free healthcare at government hospitals and subsidized care at private clinics.

"Sustainability, we see no problem as long as we do our best. And we will still continue to get external support too for research. It's a win-win situation," he said.

His sustainability plans acknowledge the fact that the folks who pioneered the IU-Kenya Partnership and then AMPATH are nearing retirement. "One of the things we are doing now is trying to follow Joe's footsteps. Bob and IU identified a replacement for Joe maybe four or five years ago," he recalled. "We need to do succession planning in all our parts so that we are able to continue. It's interesting to note that currently, the leadership is our former students. The CEO of the hospital, the dean of the school, the heads of departments."

He went on to list all the young physicians trained at Moi over the years who are now leading the institutions. There is immense pride in his voice. But he also sees challenges. "I have teams that are growing. I have several levels of consultants," he said. "I don't have a lot of the young, the very recent graduates. I'm no longer attracting them. They are into private practice very aggressively, and we are not able to catch them as easily anymore."

This is the other side of the government's hospital insurance fund that's driving the sustainability effort. "I had a gynecologist who was very good. He said, 'I do cesarean sections. What you are trying to pay me per month I can get it in one day.' He did not see why he should spend time in AMPATH."

But doctors and others at AMPATH are rewarded beyond money. "We try to downplay the money part," he said. "If you look at that [business] card I gave you, see here: 'OGW.' That's a presidential recognition—Order of the Grand Warrior of Kenya. In 2008, the then president of Kenya bestowed this on me for service to society through AMPATH."

"Amongst some of our staff, yes, they want money," he admitted. "But they still go out of their way to serve. They've seen what they have contributed to society, and that's job satisfaction. They say, 'I've worked for AMPATH,' and that gives them quite a high. It feels nice when you go to bed at night."

"When I go to the United States and speak to the Kenyan doctors living there, many of them would like to come back home, but they have no job opportunities. AMPATH has done several things. One, you can build your career here because we have a functioning clinic system. Earlier on it was HIV. Now it's population health. If you want to practice in AMPATH, you have everything you need. You have the life support. You have the expertise support. We have experts from IU and Brown and Duke and so on within reach. Any time. It is the resources here. When you have what you need to practice, you don't want to go anywhere else."

Winstone Nyandiko

Dr. Winstone Nyandiko Mokaya's office is on the second floor of the AMPATH Centre on the MTRH campus. Nyandiko is an associate professor of child health and pediatrics at Moi University as well as the director of research at AMPATH. He has been in Eldoret since becoming a tutorial fellow in 1996. He has been the executive director for research at AMPATH since 2017, but at heart he remains a pediatrician. His small office is crowded with a table and chairs—enough for a research team to meet over paperwork. The view from the window is mostly the rooftops of the hospital's older wards. But if you step out into the open hallway overlooking the central courtyard, you can almost peer into the waiting area of his pediatric comprehensive care clinic, Module 4, where children with HIV wait with their moms for their checkups. The professor does not like to be too far from his young patients.

He began our April 2019 interview by telling me about the early days of the HIV/AIDS epidemic. Before antiretroviral treatments, many mothers delivered children who were HIV positive. He had completed his mandatory preregistration medical internship at what was then Eldoret District Hospital (now MTRH) in 1994 and joined Moi University as a tutorial fellow two years later. He was on the wards during those difficult times before AMPATH secured the ARV treatment drugs that today lower the likelihood of mother-to-child transmission to almost zero.

"At the beginning, it was exhausting teaching clinical officers at rural clinics who had never known a prescription of ARVs," he recalled. "They used to be told, 'There is HIV, and it is a deadly disease. This is ARV, and it stops the transmission.' But that was not enough." Nyandiko and colleagues at the medical school were initially trained by faculty from Indiana University and other AMPATH Consortium members. Once they understood how the new drugs worked, how they were best administered, and how the therapy needed to include nutrition, care of other opportunistic infections, and general care of the family, they became the trainers. They went far afield to teach clinical officers how to deliver HIV-negative babies.

"We would be called upon to go and train in Nairobi, western Kenya, and so on. And we did a lot of trainings here at MTRH. We used to have trainings here almost twice a month just to make sure everybody was aware of what the epidemiology was, how to do adult and pediatric comprehensive care, how to do the laboratory testing, and all those things," he said. "This was a big achievement in terms of HIV care."

He recalled a long list of pediatricians trained in the early days of care, including Edith Apondi, who now heads the HIV pediatric care program and the Rafiki Centre for Excellence in Adolescent Health, also known as CCC Module 5. "There was Prof Ayaya, Prof Tenge, Dr. Nabakwe, Dr. Marete, Dr. Chumba, Dr. Gisore, Dr. Songok, and so many more," he recalled. "We learned patient care, but even it was not enough."

"We needed to know more about what we were doing to be able to investigate what was working and what could be better," he said. Many foreign universities came to Africa to do research, but they left with their findings. IU and its AMPATH Consortium were different. "They came in to be partners, not just in research, but to start with care, give us education, give us the knowledge transfer, and

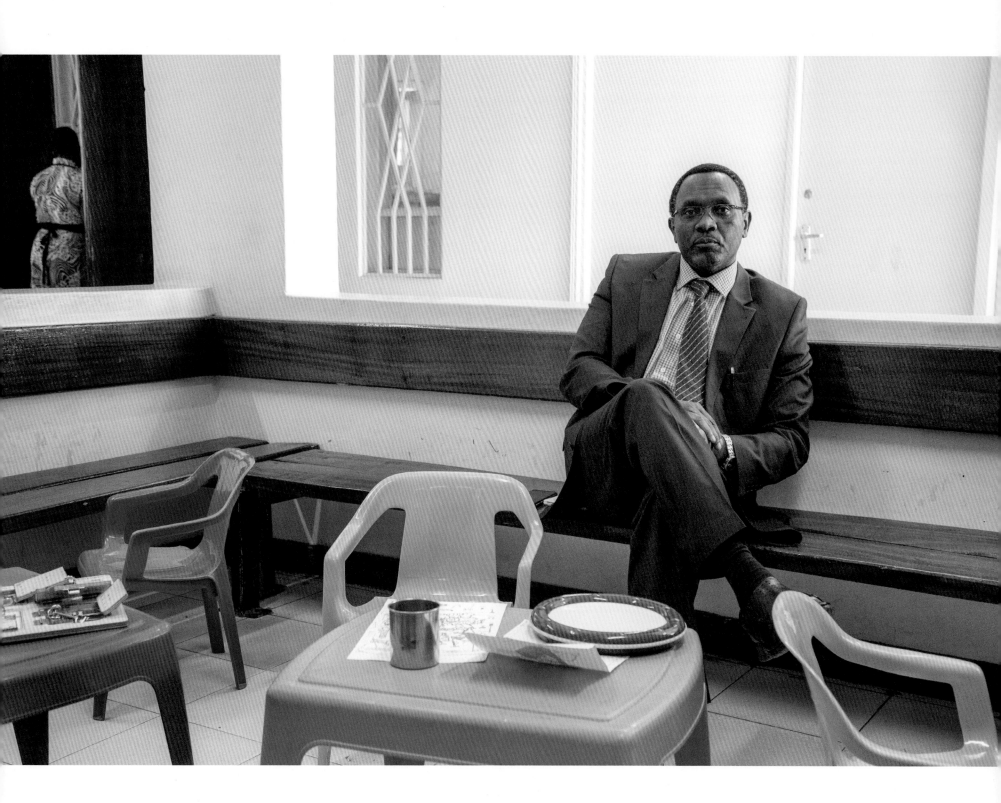

then do research in the background as they were giving service," he said. "They were always giving."

"We agreed from the onset that we must have mutual benefits to the two institutions and mutual respect for the two cultures," he continued. "You know, our cultures are very different." He used email as an example: "Here I would get an email and respond after one week. It's not that I didn't want to respond, it's just that we take time. We learned Americans wanted to be quick, so we did that," he said. "And Americans have learned to take time."

Nyandiko talked more about learning each other's culture but stressed that the collaboration was fundamentally about building capacity at a time when medical facilities were under great stress. He stated, "You are trying to develop the human resource by way of knowledge transfer and getting more people into the program, either at the technical level of doctors or at the level that can support financial management, compliance rules and regulations, and the hiring process." More than just ARVs needed to be learned. There were also medical record keeping and administration.

From the start of HIV treatment, AMPATH had stored medical records in a digital database. In the earliest days of AMPATH, forms were loaded onto PDAs, a forerunner of the computer tablets used today. That kind of computerized data collection and storage was quite a challenge in a place where electricity was unreliable and office doors and windows were usually open to the elements. But with technical expertise from Dr. Bill Tierney, then codirector of research at AMPATH who also headed a research team at the Regenstrief Institute at IU, the computerized records proved invaluable in a system where patients accessed care from multiple points and lived in places without street addresses.

"Around 2003 we were collecting so much data," Nyandiko said. "If a patient came to see me, I could use a gadget, enter the patient number to access their information, and then manage them appropriately." HIV-positive clients require a regular and consistent supply of drugs, and centralized digital records kept treatment efficient and effective.

He recalled, "Care came first, but then we said, 'Let's review what we have collected as data. What are some of the things happening in terms of outcomes?'" Nyandiko and his Moi colleagues collaborated on research studies using the data, working alongside AMPATH colleagues like Bob Einterz and Bill Tierney.

"My most exciting moments were presenting in national meetings and presenting outside the country," he said. "We traveled to Thailand for my first foreign conference. I think was in 2004 or 2005. We didn't have money for a trip like that, but Bill and Bob got us money from somewhere. And I tell you something. They put two men in the same hotel room in Thailand and we said that is not our culture! We learned so much at that meeting about treatment but also about other cultures." The Americans there were sharing rooms, so the Kenyans did too.

He explained that the current approach to research remains collaborative. "We don't encourage people to go out on their own and get an award," he said. "You look for a partner and say, 'We are going to do this, this is what we want to do,' and then of course it allows people not to have conflicts." AMPATH research efforts are parsed into several working groups that meet monthly. Each has two chairs—one Kenyan and one North American. Even Nyandiko had a codirector from the consortium: Dr. Kara Wools-Kaloustian from the IU School of Medicine.

"We also have an executive committee meeting which I cochair as the director of research on the Kenyan side. We work together from the start of an idea," he said. "I feel old, because I have worked with five different North American research leadership regimes over the years. I am looking to a point where I should be able to hand this baton to somebody else, the way I have done with pediatric HIV care. We are looking at the options of who can take this to the next level."

The professor thought back on AMPATH's long record of success in research:

> We have brought our program from one research unit to eleven. We have developed a structure supported by Moi Teaching and Referral Hospital, Moi University, and obviously the North American consortium. AMPATH has brought in knowledge transfer, they have brought in funding that built on all this infrastructure. They have been able to give us a support that allows our system to actually work. Because of the HIV care program that we built during the crisis, we have been able to have the chronic disease program we have. It has made it possible to now transition to population health and mental health. Everything now is working well.

Nyandiko slipped further into recollection. A farewell ceremony for Joe and Sarah Ellen Mamlin had been held on the MTRH graduation grounds just two weeks earlier, and the couple had left Eldoret just three days before our talk. He commented, "I can tell you that along the way, very big people made me do what I do now. Joe Mamlin is one person who everybody looks at, and I say without Joe Mamlin, a lot of things wouldn't have happened. A lot of our work etiquette and the way we deal with our patients, the seriousness of being in clinic when you are required to be there . . . we learned that from Joe. I have just now come from the clinic myself."

Indeed, Nyandiko spends a half day every week in the pediatric HIV clinic on the other side of the building from his office. He said,

> I do mentorship now. You must do mentorship because you cannot be here in perpetuity. Everyone needs to dream, to look at yourself five to ten years from now. We never used

to do that. We now even look at fifty years from now. This is a mentality which has been brought to us by our partners. I point to Joe Mamlin, John Sidle, Kara Wools-Kaloustian, Bill Tierney, Tom Inui, Rachel Vreeman, and others whom we have worked with for a long time. They brought us a lot of leadership skills. They taught us that you need to look at everything. You don't assume anything.

> When I came here in 2001, really there was nobody interested in [pediatric AIDS], and it was a killer. The overall mortality rate for infants was seventy-eight per thousand and now it has come down to about thirty-nine per thousand live births. You can imagine that huge drop, and you can imagine it is fundamentally because we took care of HIV. Right now, we are talking about transmission rate from mother to child at 2 percent. It was 20 percent when I came in the year 2000, so from the numbers alone we can see that we have made quite a bit of progress.

The children AMPATH saved in the early 2000s are now young adults. Many were born HIV positive and survived because they were prescribed ARVs in infancy. They took pills every day to keep the virus at bay, although most didn't know why until they were in their early teens. "The biggest story is around our children we were able to save. Children I was seeing then at two years old are now in their twenties and healthy and going about their business and going to school. One of them is actually a medical student in Maseno," Nyandiko said proudly, referring to the Maseno School of Medicine, Kenya's newest medical school located just seventy-five miles southwest of Eldoret.

"You talk to those guys and you feel nice. These days, when I go to the clinic and meet these young children and their mothers and we are talking and you are giving them hope and you are giving disclosure [telling them why they take pills]," he said. At fourteen years of age, children are transferred to a special clinic specifically for adolescents—the Rafiki Centre, which means "friends" in Swahili. He continued, "We never used to have Rafiki, but now we are able to transition them after disclosure to a clinic where they are able to meet and share and motivate each other. It is big. You feel that you have achieved something in your life which is really important."

I asked Nyandiko why he stays in Eldoret when he has been to Harvard for a Master of Public Health degree and knows he could go back to the US and have an easier life. "I think the first thing is really around the way we have built our partnership. All of our partners have had the same characteristic. They come and they don't impose things on us. We are mutual. We become true partners. We look for equity," he explained. "For me, the second most important thing is seeing a person come from the US, who comes to the ground and calls this home and settles in and helps Kenyans. You ask yourself, if he can come from outside and stay here, get dirt on his boots and dirt on his hands, why should I who has benefited from the Kenyan taxpayer in training, who has benefited from this collaboration, go and go away?"

"I would rather be inside trying to work things out from inside rather than run to the outside," he explained. "Now my biggest joy is the fact that what we started as a single, HIV-based program called the Academic Model for the Prevention and Treatment of HIV is now an Academic Model for Providing Access to Healthcare. It is not just around patient care. It is about structure. It is about attitude. It is about culture. It is about making sure you are leaving a generation of people who can take over."

Jeremiah Laktabai

Dr. Jeremiah Laktabai has never quite been able to leave the rural town of Webuye, population 19,600. I first met him in the office of chief of party Sylvester Kimaiyo on the top floor of the AMPATH Centre. He was filling in while his boss was at meetings in Nairobi. The office was familiar to him since the AMPATH leadership meets there regularly and because he has been a protégé of Kimaiyo since the early years of the epidemic. He does not usually sit in at the chief's desk, however.

Laktabai is one of two leaders at AMPATH who oversee the new population health initiative, a project that proposes to upend the traditional disease model that has so long driven healthcare decisions. The focus is on prevention. He said, "We know people need to access healthcare when they are unwell, but we also know that disease just doesn't appear out of thin air. Disease takes a journey. It can sometimes be prevented, can be arrested, can be modified at some lower level," long before most people seek a doctor's care. But in the Kenyan setting, "there are many issues that go hand in hand with health and disease and wellness. The socioeconomic determinants of health are hugely relevant." Poverty precludes the early interventions that Laktabai and his colleagues see as key to providing the kind of medical care that prevents illness before a cure is necessary.

"We could have the best inventions at a high level," he stated—like the kind the tertiary care hospital in Eldoret provides—"but if intervention is not reaching the person out in the village who needs it most, then we remain an academic high tower." Laktabai doesn't want to live in a high tower. He wants to provide care to every Kenyan who needs it, and he wants to provide that care at the earliest stages.

I asked why he thought population health was the correct approach to meeting Kenya's healthcare needs. "Because this is how we deliver to the village level," he answered. And most of Kenya lives in the village. "Care happens here in the dialysis center of the MTRH, but

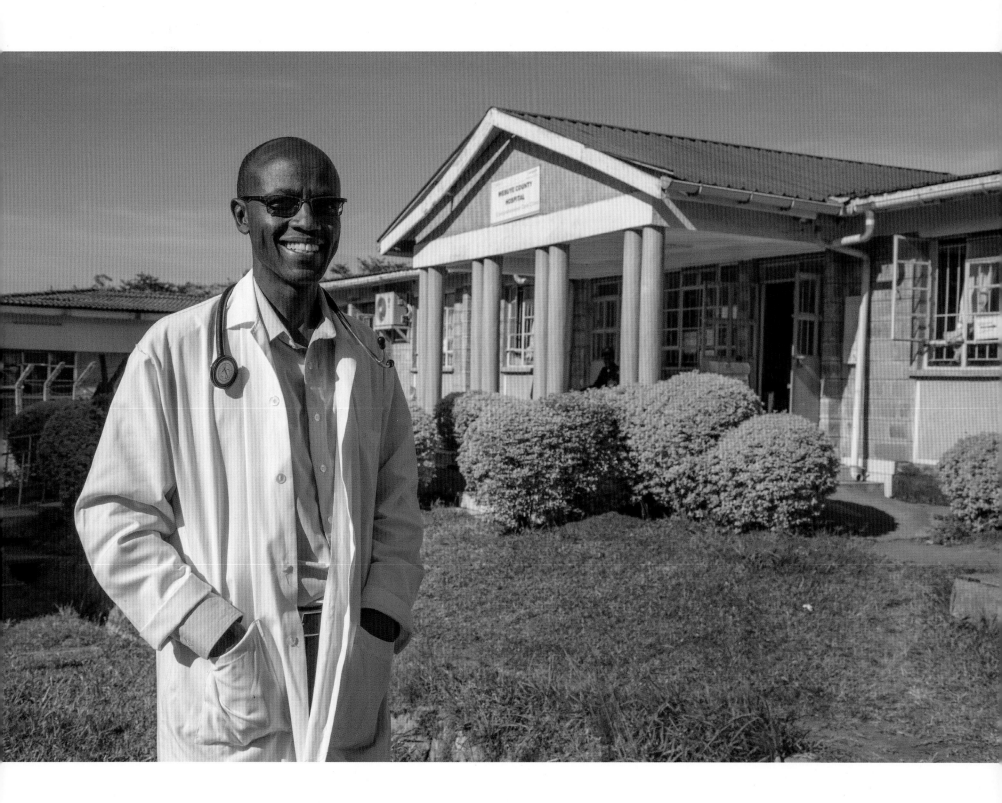

that's the tip of the pyramid. It is at the base where care is most needed, and that base is in the village."

For Laktabai, that theoretical village could well be somewhere near Webuye, an industrial town in Bungoma County on the main road to Uganda, about thirty-five miles west of Eldoret. The town houses a chemical factory, a sugar factory, and a huge paper factory building that was shuttered a dozen years ago. For miles and miles around, though, there are villages of subsistence farmers who go to the Webuye County Hospital when they are too sick to work and beyond the expertise of the village dispensary. The hospital is a clinical training site for the Moi University family medicine program and serves a catchment area of about one hundred thousand people. Laktabai is there every week. It is how he keeps in touch with the base of the pyramid.

It was mid-April when he picked me up from my house near the MTRH. I rode with him in his Toyota sedan for one of his weekly visits to the Webuye hospital. The dry season was nearing its end. The corn fields we drove past had been harvested weeks earlier. At one point just past Leseru, a dozen grey crowned cranes pecked at grain left in the field just fifty feet from the roadside. Each stood a yard tall with a crown of stiff golden feathers on its head. Western tourists would have stopped the car. We headed straight for Webuye.

"We now understand that food and income security is a major component of health," he explained. He said that people ask, "Can I afford to pay for my food, can I afford to pay for my transportation, for my children's school fees, for my healthcare?" He sees great potential in the land. Most people in western Kenya have a small plot of land. They have resources that, with a little support in the form of education and technical assistance, could generate an excess of food. According to Laktabai, "At that point, you get to save some money, and you can use it to buy insurance. You get to protect the little that you have from a catastrophic event. And that event is usually a single hospitalization. You know, it just flattens a whole family's resources."

The National Hospital Insurance Fund figures prominently in the population health model. NHIF is a government-owned corporation with a mandate to provide health insurance to all Kenyans over the age of eighteen. It started in 1967 but until recently has been largely restricted to the formal sector of the economy—the folks who get regular paychecks. But the informal sector of subsistence farmers and day workers makes up the bulk of the country's workers. In 2014, the Kenya National Bureau of Statistics estimated that the informal sector represented 82.7 percent of employment.

In the wake of the postelection violence of 2008, Kenya drafted and ratified a new national constitution, replacing the one first written at independence in 1963. Among its many reforms, the 2010 constitution "devolved" power from the central government in Nairobi to a new system of forty-seven semiautonomous counties headed by local governors and included a legal framework to ensure a comprehensive, rights-based approach to healthcare. In 2017, President Kenyatta announced that the country would achieve funding for universal healthcare via the NHIF for both the formal and informal sectors. NHIF is therefore seen as the mechanism that will pay for universal health. The key is getting people to buy it.

"AMPATH and the government are on the same page," he said, and then he continued,

Over the past few months, we have had an opportunity to offer education and an opportunity to enroll people in insurance at the household level. We have done house-to-house visits to over two thousand households. It's interesting that people are eager for healthcare insurance. They are willing and they are ready to embrace this insurance.

When we started, we thought that maybe a small percentage of people would be excited about it, but to know that people are willing and ready to sign up, that people do care for their health . . . They are willing to pay 500 shillings per month [US$5] once you fill in the gaps for them.

The gaps he refers to are largely knowledge gaps. Laktabai said, "People in the villages don't know how a health insurance product works. It has been interesting to see the village elders and assistant chiefs and chiefs take to the idea once they understand it. They say, 'In my area this is the thing that we need. Our families say yes, we are going to do this. Just make sure that the healthcare is there for us.'"

He slowed the car as we approached the town of Turbo because he knew there was often a police car with a radar gun there. He's been nabbed a few times over the years. Sometimes the good doctor is given a pass because even the police appreciate their doctors. But sometimes he has to pay a KSh 20,000 (US$200) fine to the courts. He says it's worth it to get back to Webuye.

Ten years earlier, Laktabai had been the medical superintendent at Webuye Hospital. As an administrator, he had struggled with the limitations of a developing economy. "I had to worry about firewood and beans. You know, we have to have beans for the patients' meals and firewood to cook them with," he recalled. "Then all of a sudden, we'd say, 'Ooh, guys, there is no electricity!'" Laktabai knew that government funding was insufficient but also knew that patients would pay for good service.

"Healthcare can bring in money, especially when there is NHIF," he said. "Good service generates income." He learned this by listening to the community. AMPATH succeeded because it looked to the community for solutions from the beginning. In his words, "What is this thing that the community needs, and what is this thing that can work for the community?"

According to Laktabai, AMPATH is "woven into the life of the Kenyan. You can't really say, 'Let's remove AMPATH.' You can't really say, 'Let's dissect this AMPATH, pull it out, and then the other [parts] will continue.' I think the philosophy of Leading with Care has been like the HIV virus that gets into the blood system and the only way to kill the virus is to kill the person." It is a strange analogy, but in a place where HIV is a lifelong reality for so many, it speaks to the tenacity of the philosophy and the dedication of AMPATH's workers to community care.

I asked what motivates him and his team of healthcare workers beyond this slogan. He said, "I think it is the realization that we can make a difference. Actually, there is so much to do. But even in the midst of epidemic, there is something that can be done, and there is a system that is responsive to what needs to be done. You realize, yes, not just that it ought to be happening but that I can participate in."

In a poor country with so many challenges, AMPATH's success at stemming the HIV epidemic is a clear and certain success. "Wow, look at that, we have worked together and this has happened!" he said. "That is the thing which says, 'Let's do the next thing.' Because everywhere you can see a change, you can see an influence on attitude. You can see the program bearing fruits, and the fruit is sweet."

"You see the chronic disease burden and you realize that it is so familiar to the HIV burden, and we say, 'Yes, we should be able to do something about it,'" he said. "It's like, 'Yes, such can be addressed. A functioning system has been created.'"

Laktabai pointed to the system of community health volunteers (CHVs) as key to that functioning system. Hundreds of people living in the villages have been trained by AMPATH to visit their neighbors and look for signs of illness. At the beginning of the HIV epidemic, the focus was entirely on testing for the virus and providing support to positive people. Now the CHVs monitor the health of people in their villages on a range of chronic illnesses, including breast and cervical cancer, tuberculosis, diabetes, hypertension, and so on. They inform medical staff at the local dispensaries or the county hospital about local health issues before they become overwhelming. And lately, they have been explaining how NHIF works and encouraging subscription. For those 500 shillings, all the care needed by the entire family is covered, whether at the dispensary, the county hospital, or even a referral to the MTRH in Eldoret.

Laktabai makes the weekly visit to Webuye so he can do rounds with the local doctors, check in on difficult patients, and joke around with the staff. In a way, his clinical day serves AMPATH almost as if the good doctor was himself a CHV. He is reminded of the challenges encountered by a county hospital and the extraordinary dedication required for care at that level. "They say the more the school, the less the availability," he said. "I think our collaboration has changed that. Like-minded, transformative leaders with a similar vision of community care have turned that idea around."

Population health is a big idea that will require leaders to engage the community at the village level all across Kenya. It is why Laktabai visits Webuye every week. And it is why he is so often sitting in the chief of party's office.

Wilson Aruasa

Dr. Wilson Kipkirui Aruasa is one of the newer members of the AMPATH leadership. He began as CEO of the MTRH in 2016, but he is a product of the long partnership between his hospital and Moi University. He earned his undergraduate degree at Moi and spent more than ten years at MTRH as the director of clinical services and then another six years as deputy CEO before taking the top position. He now directs the daily operation of one of Kenya's two public referral hospitals, a one-thousand-bed tertiary academic medical center serving a population of approximately twenty-four million in western Kenya.

I met him in his office on the top floor of the Chandaria Centre. Floor-to-ceiling windows form a ninety-degree arch of glass with views of Nandi Road and the medical school on the other side. "When I moved in, the windows were covered with drapes," he said as I sat down to talk with him on a couple of overstuffed chairs on either side of a small glass table. "As you can see, I had them taken down so that I could see people and also so that people could see that I am here."

At MTRH, Moi University School of Medicine students and residents, together with students from consortium member universities, get practical, hands-on experience. The medical campus includes the AMPATH Centre and several specialty care buildings including the Chandaria Cancer and Chronic Diseases Centre, the Riley Mother Baby Hospital, the Shoe4Africa Children's Hospital, the Rafiki Centre for Excellence in Adolescent Health, and the Majaliwa Surgical Center.

Aruasa speaks fondly of the education he received at Moi. "As a medical student, I interacted with many visiting lecturers from Indiana University as well as many medical students and nursing students coming from Indiana and other medical schools in the AMPATH Consortium," he said. By the time he had his degree and returned from a residency in Busia on the Ugandan border in 2001, Joe Mamlin, whom he had met back in 1993, was back in Eldoret, and the AMPATH Consortium was in full operation. "He and I used to work in the medical outpatient clinic and on the wards together," he recalled. "I went to Indiana University in 2008 to do a course on health information management at the Regenstrief Institute for

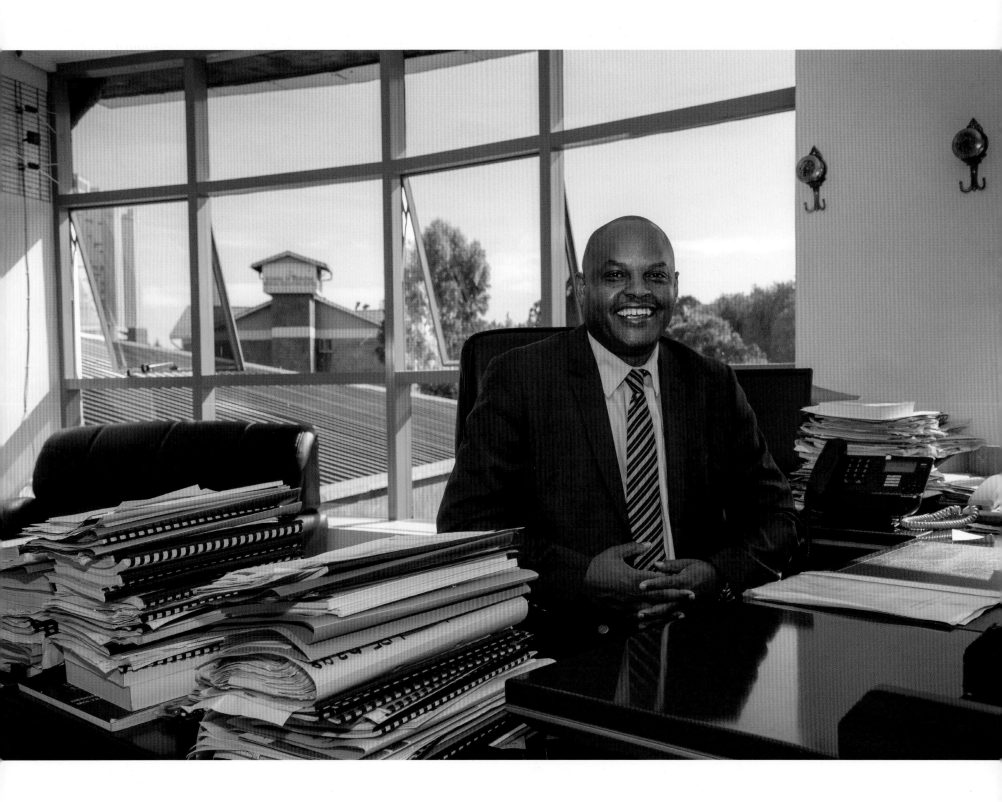

about two months." Bill Tierney and Dr. Tim Mercer, an AMPATH medicine team leader, helped him understand US health systems, and he became increasingly interested in hospital administration.

"I've met great people in the program, including Bob Einterz, who has been the key leader from the Indiana side, and I've met many other people from Duke University, from Brown University, from University of Toronto in Canada, and many others," he said. He said that by 2009, "We were transforming [the HIV operation] into the Academic Model Providing Access to Healthcare. We were going beyond HIV/AIDS and into the full spectrum of care, particularly chronic diseases, and even to primary healthcare issues about water and sanitation, issues about food safety and security."

He continued, "Now I sit on the executive committee of AMPATH, which meets regularly every month with the purpose of reviewing the work of the management and the research grants and also the care program. I also chair the AMPATH Board, which alternates between the Moi University principal of the College of Health Sciences and my office."

Aruasa sees two primary reasons the collaboration among his hospital, the university, and the consortium has succeeded. "First of all, it is the model itself. It is a model whereby North American institutions have made two primarily Kenyan institutions work together. That is Moi University and Moi Teaching and Referral Hospital," he explained.

> You see, the way it is in Kenya is that institutions stand alone. You will find a Moi University. They would say they are in the Ministry of Education and that they have nothing to do with Moi Teaching and Referral Hospital, which is in the Ministry of Health. IU brought the two institutions together. To me, the collaboration of Moi University,

Moi Teaching and Referral Hospital, and the consortium of American institutions led by Indiana University is the biggest factor that has made AMPATH work. It is what I am proudest of. Working together collaboratively in a team effort has been the biggest factor in the success of AMPATH. And it is not just the institutions per se, it is also the individuals.

He talked of "individuals like Bob Einterz and Joe Mamlin and Sarah Ellen Mamlin, Adrian Gardner, Tom Inui, John Sidle, and Bill Tierney. All of them have been pillars of the AMPATH success, as well as very strong individuals from the University of Toronto and from Duke University." He continued, "Some have come and spent time in Eldoret to teach and to do research with us. All those strong individuals who are committed and passionate. They have contributed a lot."

"And alongside them we have had leaders like Prof Fabian Esamai, Prof Paul Ayuo, and Prof Lukoye Atwoli. To me those have been very great pillars of the institution," he explained. "And in MTRH we have Prof Kimaiyo, Prof Nyandiko, plus Robert Rono and Christine Chuani who work in the RSPO, and, of course, Prof Mengech who started it all," he concluded.

Haroun Mengech was the founding dean of Moi University's medical school and later the CEO of MTRH. As dean, he set a clear mandate that learning medicine required the practice of medicine in the villages, since that was where most Kenyans lived. Mengech himself had grown up in rural Nandi County just south of Eldoret. The core of the new school's curriculum was a community-based experience and service (COBES) program where, from the start of coursework to the end, students spent a portion of their time in nearby village clinics. This experiential approach differed dramatically from the one Mengech himself had studied under at the University of

Nairobi, where the first two years of medical school were entirely theoretical. Students spent most of their time memorizing things rather than thinking for themselves and solving practical problems. His school would educate doctors who could treat patients effectively but could also analyze the healthcare environment and propose solutions for the challenges that affected the community where the care was being delivered.

Aruasa said, "These leaders brought us to a point in time where we are looking beyond curing diseases and looking at prevention. We are looking at the population health model where we try to see that every person in the community has access to health insurance, even when they are well. Should they get the need to go for treatment, they should not be exposed financially." The CEO credits the Ministry of Health for having supported the AMPATH collaboration over the years and, now, for working with it to make national healthcare sustainable though expansion of the National Hospital Insurance Fund, a national health insurance plan that promises to make quality healthcare affordable and available to all fifty million Kenyans within the decade.

He also credits the Research and Sponsored Projects Office as key to the acceptance of the uniquely strong partnership among the three institutions. "That office has been very instrumental in the success of AMPATH because it plays the administrative and financial management role that is key to any institution," said Aruasa. "Because we have RSPO, all administrative issues, including procurement, staff issues, staff salaries, donor funding, NIH funding, and USAID funding, are managed well." This is Aruasa's very diplomatic way of saying that RSPO has always operated without the corruption that weakens and even defeats so many institutions in his country. This high level of accountability and transparency in

accounting and administration at MTRH is sadly rare in Africa, but it is certainly a huge reason so many transnational medical and pharmaceutical companies have worked with AMPATH and MTRH for so long.

"There's another person that I cannot talk about without saying his name—Eli Lilly. For the last fifteen years, the Lilly Endowment, whose headquarters are in Indianapolis, has given us medications of all kinds: for cancer, for mental health, and for diabetes. All this to the tune of KSh 20 billion or US$200 million per year. As we speak now, we are awaiting another consignment being shipped from Indiana. Those medicines not only help patients in MTRH but in the whole western half of Kenya. Millions of people have been benefitted for free because of that support," he said.

Dozens of other corporate foundations have contributed medicines and other therapies to AMPATH, including Abbott Fund, AbbVie, AstraZeneca, Boehringer Ingelheim, Bristol Myers Squibb, Celgene, Corteva Agriscience, Merck, Pfizer, and Takeda. The virtually unblemished financial management record that MTRH, Moi University, and AMPATH together have built over the decades underpins a work environment that encourages loyalty and longevity.

I had heard Joe Mamlin, Adrian Gardner, and others claim that the length of tenure for trained medical staff—doctors, nurses, technicians, and others—is far longer than one would expect given the "brain drain" in Africa. The World Health Organization (WHO) reports that Africa bears more than 24 percent of the global burden of disease but has access to only 3 percent of health workers. Kenya has just one doctor per five thousand Kenyans, five times higher than the WHO minimum acceptable physician-to-population ratio of one per one thousand (Ighobor 2017). Part of the problem is insufficient supply and part is the "brain drain," where physicians and other medical practitioners leave the country for better pay and working conditions in the UK, the US, and Australia. Even though Kenya's big medical schools in Eldoret and Nairobi graduate about six hundred doctors each year, and newer medical schools at Kenyatta, Egerton, and Maseno universities are now beginning to graduate doctors too, hundreds and hundreds of Kenya's doctors nevertheless leave the country each year.

Aruasa proudly points to the high retention rates at MTRH. "If we take the 'big cats' like doctors, right now retention is almost 100 percent," he said. "Nurses is where we have a retention rate of about 95 percent. And the reason for this is that nurses tend to get better-paying jobs in the US and Australia. The rest of the staff who are not doctors and not nurses, that's another 100 percent. None of them ever quit," he concluded, because working at MTRH is a good job.

I asked about statistics at other hospitals in Kenya. "I know in private hospitals and some other government hospitals, for doctors it could probably be 60, 70 percent retention. They keep looking either outside the country, looking to MTRH, or looking at another institution similar to MTRH," he explained. "Nurses are very fluid. In the counties, retention is probably just about 70 percent. A lot leave for US and Australia—a lot more than it happens in MTRH," he said, noting that loss of trained medical personnel to the West is a real strain on resources.

"The role of AMPATH in staff retention ranks very high. It gives people a different perspective to their work. It gives a variety of influences," he said. "Most CEOs would only work as a CEO in the hospital. But here at MTRH, I am also involved in research. I am involved with the population health initiative. I am involved in providing primary healthcare. That's not common for a CEO."

"I tell you, Prof, it is most important to have individuals who are committed and passionate. Those are the ones who that have made the difference and will make the difference going forward," he continued. "This country is transforming. We are now working on what government calls the Big Four agenda. One of them is universal health coverage by expanding the national hospital insurance registration [NHIF]," he explained. "But MTRH and AMPATH were always ahead. Even before government thought about that, we have been turning people to NHIF since 2008. We were ten years ahead of the rest of the country, and now, through the population health initiative and the work of the medical and social work departments of MTRH, we are even accelerating it so that we get more healthy people to have insurance."

He added, "And I will tell you, if I look at it ten years back in MTRH, when a patient was admitted in the general side of the hospital, chances were that the patient had no insurance cover. Today, based on the latest statistics that I've seen, 35 to 40 percent have the NHIF cover. Which is very high. I mean it's higher than the national average by probably 10 percent. NHIF is the path to population health."

Aruasa had helped organize the goodbye celebration for Joe and Sarah Ellen Mamlin on the graduation grounds of the MTRH a few weeks earlier. A thousand people at the MTRH had turned out to celebrate the Mamlins before they headed to Indiana for retirement. "Joe said he will be happy when the population health is successful. That is our focus now, and I want to assure you that that MTRH is going to play its role to make sure that the population health is successful," Arusa said.

Aruasa's optimism springs from a medical education based on community service and care. It has been nourished by study in North America sponsored by universities in the AMPATH Consortium and sustained by the continuing collaboration of Moi University, the Ministry of Health, and the many AMPATH doctors who, like Joe Mamlin, come to Eldoret and make lifelong friendships with him.

Laura Ruhl

Dr. Laura Ruhl is a child of AMPATH. She first visited Kenya as an undergraduate student in an anthropology class at Washington University in the summer of 2000. "I learned my Swahili then and fell in love with Kenya. I fell in love with the diversity of culture, the landscape, and kind of every aspect of life here. I knew when I finished that course that I wanted to come back," she recalled.

And she has come back to Kenya—many times. On the day of her interview, Laura was the field director for Population Health, just one of the many titles she has had since first visiting Kenya. As codirector with her longtime Kenyan colleague, Jeremiah Laktabai, she led AMPATH's newest and most ambitious initiative—providing universal healthcare to all Kenyans. To understand how this happened, I asked her how she got to Eldoret the first time and why she kept coming back.

During the year between graduating university and starting medical school, Laura had worked in neighboring Uganda on a "safe motherhood" project funded by USAID that focused on child health and reduction of maternal mortality. While living in the capital, Kampala, she researched medical schools back home where she could earn a degree that would prepare her for work in the developing world. She chose Indiana University because of AMPATH. "I went directly from Uganda into medical school, which was a really difficult transition," she said. "I sat down immediately with Bob Einterz and said, 'I'm going to be a Slemenda scholar,' and he said, 'Well, here's an application form.'"

Slemenda scholarships are very competitive. They were developed in 1998 to help rising second-year medical students gain experience in global health by working with AMPATH. Slemenda scholars attend classes at Moi University, make rounds in the MTRH, work with ongoing field projects conducted by AMPATH faculty, and live with Kenyan medical students in the dormitory (hostel) during their time in Eldoret. Only two are awarded most years. Laura landed one, just as she had told Bob she would.

"That first year of medical school was incredibly challenging. I almost dropped out at one point," she said, but the promise of going back to Kenya impelled her, and the scholarship made it possible. She arrived in Eldoret in the summer of 2003. AMPATH was then treating hundreds of HIV-positive patients and managing larger and larger donations from abroad. But the AIDS epidemic was still raging, and all medical staff were under incredible stress. Sarah Ellen Mamlin was back home visiting Indiana when Laura arrived, so Joe Mamlin was all alone as he welcomed Laura back to Kenya.

"We students were staying up at the student hostel across the street from MTRH. We spent a lot of time on the hospital wards observing," she recalled. "It was then that I first saw Joe sit down with patients. He was doing some experimental work on preventing mother-to-child transmission. I learned so much about making a personal connection with patients." Joe and his Kenyan colleagues taught by engaging students with patients on a near-daily basis.

On the weekends, Joe, Laura, and the other students from the US would go on excursions together, and her affection for the old doctor grew. "I saw the beginning of the

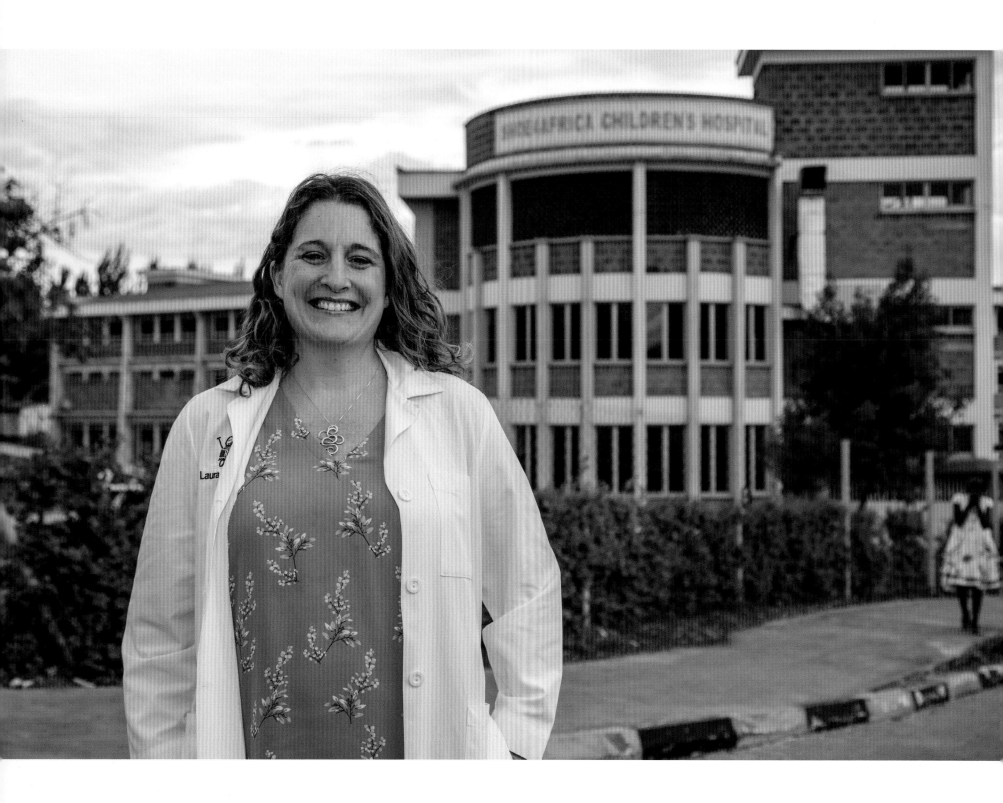

response to AIDS that summer. It was all being done very quietly because stigma was so bad then." Indeed, though drugs were available and thousands were being treated, most people in western Kenya still thought of HIV as a death sentence. They did not yet understand the virus, but they knew its history, and it was terrifying.

"By the time I came back as a fourth-year medical student in December 2005, a huge transformation had taken place. AMPATH had PEPFAR funding from USAID and was treating thousands of HIV-positive patients," she said. "I got to work on the PMTCT [prevention of mother-to-child transmission of HIV] program. I got to team up with the intern and have a truly clinical experience." The dramatic decrease in infant mortality brought on by the PMTCT program had done much to reduce the fear of AIDS locally, and AMPATH's treatment and public education programs had greatly decreased stigma.

"By the end of the rotation, I knew I wanted to go into global health, but I felt I needed to try a different program since I had spent so much time in Eldoret," she said. "I went to Minnesota and did a global health residency. I went to Thailand briefly but came back because I wanted to keep the door open for doing the team leadership position at AMPATH." Her plan worked. She got the leadership slot. "But even after coming to Eldoret as team leader in 2010, I still thought I needed to go somewhere else. I knew AMPATH, and I loved AMPATH, and I knew AMPATH was doing the right thing, but I felt like it was important to get different perspectives."

So, after another year in Eldoret, she went back to the US to get a master's degree in public health at the University of North Carolina. She worked with some global health programs in the states, but by 2017, she was back again living full time in Eldoret and teaching at Moi. "I just couldn't find a program that embodied everything that AMPATH did," she said. "None of [the other programs] had as much collaboration within university departments as did IU and Moi, let alone collaboration among multiple universities like the AMPATH Consortium. I concluded that AMPATH's focus on collaboration—whether it was between North American universities or between Moi's medical school and the referral hospital in Eldoret—was something truly unique. It's often messy, and there's lots of drama sometimes, but it's much easier to get things done when people are talking and working together."

I asked Laura why AMPATH has succeeded. She replied,

> It's relationships. There's a lot of respect between colleagues. I respect them. They respect me. We have disagreements, but we don't allow things to fall apart because there is that respect. We North Americans are not here just to benefit ourselves. We really are here to develop our colleagues and to learn from them. We are now at a point where many of my Kenyan colleagues have more skills than I have. We are at a point where together we can create a system where Kenyans who are poor or otherwise unable to access healthcare can get quality care. Even if people are pulled in many, many directions, everyone does have the same goal.

She described one point of tension, saying, "Oftentimes North Americans here are able to commit 100 percent of their time to the work of AMPATH. Kenyans are pulled in many different directions, however. They have responsibilities that we don't have. We North Americans are always visitors here. We try to keep that in mind, though it is difficult because for many of us, Kenya is our home too."

The house she then called home had been the home of another Hoosier until just a few days earlier. For nearly twenty years, Joe and Sarah Ellen Mamlin had lived in

Facing, As a pediatrician, Laura Ruhl frequently rounds in the Shoe4Africa Children's Hospital on the MTRH campus. It is the only public hospital for children in East Africa. She codirects the Population Health initiative for the AMPATH Consortium and is an assistant professor of clinical medicine at the IU School of Medicine in Indianapolis. Her first visit to Kenya was in 2000 as an undergraduate university student. She now lives in the Mamlins' old house with her husband, Matt Turissini, and their daughters.

the beautiful house where Laura and I sat, surrounded by trellised bougainvillea, frangipani trees, and playground toys. Laura had visited with the Mamlins in this home more times that she could count, but now it was her house. She said it still felt a little strange. She and her husband, Matt Turissini, a medical team leader at AMPATH, slept in the Mamlins' bedroom, and their two daughters slept in rooms that had earlier hosted Mamlin children and family guests over the years. They ate their meals at the table on which the Mamlins had so often spread out provisions. They held Thursday happy hour parties and invited friends into the yard where Sarah Ellen and Joe only a month earlier had sat and watched Laura and Tim's children play.

She and I were talking while sheltered by the roof of a small, wall-less hut in the front yard that Laura and Matt had only a day before decided to call "Joe's banda." She told me she had sat in my chair and talked with Joe many times during the sixteen years she had been leaving and returning to Eldoret.

It was clear that Eldoret was a special place for Laura, so I asked if its charms are the real reason for AMPATH's success. She replied, "I think it is something that could have happened anywhere in the world. I don't think it's Eldoret or specifically Kenya. I think it is that people here have been empowered. They have seen improvements and seen patients reclaim their dignity as well as their health. They have now worked within a fully functioning health system. They now have a better job satisfaction, better personal income, better personal growth, and they have created a new normal. Continuing to grow this healthcare system is just what's expected now. There are so many benefits from what has been created."

She continued, "I think that's especially true of the middle cadre of AMPATH workers—they want to stay here because things are good for them. Where it gets more difficult is for the Ministry of Health workers who are not part of AMPATH because they are straddling the university and the MoH, and there remain some negative aspects that can wear on you."

"I have watched my colleague Julia Songok [head of pediatrics at Moi University] totally pull out of AMPATH activities because her administrative appointment is sucking the life out of her. She's extremely dedicated, willing to do the best of her abilities, and she will never give up. If she was somewhere else in a similar situation, she might just leave, but here, she cares and knows things can be improved," Laura explained. "We have tried to get her fellowships abroad, but she says, 'I want to be in Eldoret,' and it's because of her time with AMPATH."

Lots of Laura's Kenyan colleagues stay because they are building their country, but I ask Laura why she has devoted so much of her life to Eldoret and AMPATH. "I would like to tell you that it is our patients who motivate us, but I don't think it is, at least not for me. It is more the relationships I have it with my colleagues and feeling a sense of responsibility for what we began together. I don't want to abandon that and just be a visitor," she said. "We started something, and it is good. And we are going to get it done. Even if I leave and am gone for years, I will come back. I will figure out how to weave it into my career in the future. There are so many of us who have managed to do that. The collaboration of so many universities allows medical personnel like me to return again and again."

While she said it is her devotion to colleagues that keeps her coming back, that is not to say Eldoret doesn't have a special appeal. "Physically, it's kind of like the best place you could ever live. It's perfect temperatures; not hot, not cold. Beautiful landscape. It's green. You get these gorgeous rains. The wildlife. The bird life. It's just very alive. It's the ideal spot to live. I think the loveliness of Kenya influences people, but I don't think that's the big pull."

The big pull is the work, the collaboration, and the mission, she says. So, I ask how the population health project fits into the mission for her. Laura explained, "My involvement with population health just came naturally for me. I went into internal medicine and pediatrics because I could never seem to choose a singular focus. I liked studying across the life span, so I broadened my training into preventative medicine. I was perfectly situated to think both about upstream social determinants of health, as well as how it interrelates with clinical medicine." She continued,

> I think what's become clear to me in the last six months is that population health is the vision for AMPATH. We want to increase cohesiveness between programs and within the care system. We want to figure out how to finance it and improve economics within our communities. But how do you enact that vision when you have at least fifty programs within AMPATH, each with their own funding mechanisms and management structures? Well, now we have a vision, we have a map, and we have a plan to get everyone to buy into the vision. Operationalizing that vision is really challenging, but we can do it.

"The county governments are taking on so much more responsibly for health under devolution," she said. Devolution has been ongoing since Kenya passed a new constitution in 2010 that shifts more and more responsibility for governance from Nairobi out to the forty-seven counties. Where once county hospitals and clinics reported to the capital and received funding based on formulas and national policies, now medical administrations increasingly report to county officials who decide how to allocate the tax money that supports the healthcare system. Everyone I talked with while in Kenya thought that devolution was working to the benefit of ordinary people and had decreased corruption, but other national efforts in the battle against corruption were having adverse effects on the way the AMPATH Consortium could run.

"I think there are a lot of questions on the horizon. But what is clear is that even if those of us who live here long term left tomorrow, AMPATH would continue. That might even be the biggest sign of success," she said with a bit of melancholy. "When the daily need for North American inputs is no longer there, we will have worked ourselves out of the job we wanted to work ourselves out of. It is unsettling. This is our home. We love it here. We don't want to leave. But that's the goal, right? It is a Kenyan-led program now, and that's what it should be."

"This is been my home for a long time. Matt and I met here, I came here two weeks after my wedding, seven months pregnant, so I have put down some roots here," she said. The couple recently bought a house in Indiana, just in case the time to leave Kenya comes sooner than hoped for. The "Ruhlissinis," as Laura and Tim like to call their family, love Kenya but know that someday they, like Joe and Sarah Ellen, will return to the US for good. The Kenyans are indeed taking over.

Julia Songok

Dr. Julia Songok is a child of AMPATH—somewhat like her close friend Laura Ruhl, but not exactly. "I was born here. My home, Lessos, is just a one-hour drive south of Eldoret," she explained. "I studied both medical school and residency here. I am a child of AMPATH, yes. But a Kenyan child." Julia began medical school in 1993, just a few months after the country's first multiparty elections since independence thirty years earlier. The ethnic

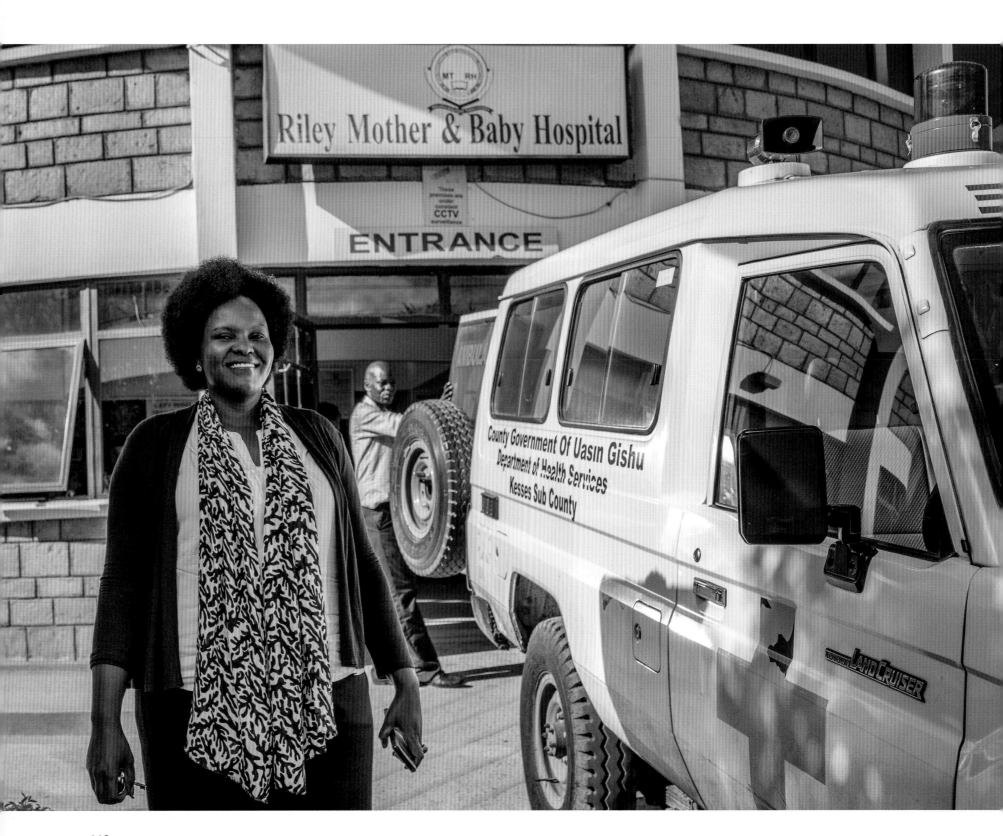

violence that followed in the Great Rift Valley still hung in the air. Julia's was just the third class of Moi students, and the radical approach to education initiated by the Moi University Faculty of Health Sciences was still unproven.

When I sat down with her in her MTRH office, she was a department head leading eleven faculty physicians in the Moi University School of Medicine. Not long before, she was coleading an AMPATH initiative called Chama cha MamaToto (collaborative mother-baby groups), with groups that focus village women's attention on health education and leverage mutually supportive relationships among women raising children. The professor has all three of her degrees from Moi: a Bachelor of Medicine, a Bachelor of Surgery, and a Master of Medicine in child health and pediatric medicine. The instruction centered on a hands-on, community-level educational approach where students were challenged to come up with answers to tough questions. Such was not always the Kenyan way of learning. "When we came here as one of the pioneer classes, education at Moi was very different from what we'd known before. It was not a subtle difference. It was stark. It was strange," she said. "It was so unlike our primary school and high school, which was very lecture based. Someone stood and told you what to think, what to understand, what do, and what to read."

Haroun Mengech, the first dean of the new medical school, had rejected the lecture-dominated pedagogy common at the University of Nairobi and other medical schools in the former colonial universities of East Africa. He had arrived in Eldoret in 1990 with what academics now refer to as an experiential learning pedagogy. Students would learn by doing at his new school, and they would learn where most Africans lived—in the villages.

"When we joined medical school, we studied the basic sciences, but you were also literally plunked into the clinical area and shown how to relate what you were seeing on the wards to what you were learning in those basic sciences," she said. "You were not just sitting there studying anatomy, physiology, biochemistry, microbiology without having a patient in mind."

"You began to really see the relationship between the patient and the science, right through and through," she continued. "There was also a lot of small group discussions that encouraged problem-based learning. You might start a microbiology class talking about a patient who has an infection. Not just saying, 'These diagrams show negatives and such.' No, you had to read through a problem that said, 'This patient came with this problem and has been unwell for this long, and these are the symptoms and signs. He's gone to see a doctor and had some tests done, and so on.'"

According to her, "This then opened it up to a discussion about the basic sciences that applied and then all the clinical things that needed to happen around that patient. And it was never just a medical problem, it was a community problem. And it was not just a community problem, it was a lab challenge. It was always something that started with the practical components and then opened up from there."

"We had to shift our thinking completely. We had to think about a problem and examine the learning objectives in the underlying issues," she recalled. "Right from first year, you had to go house to house and talk to people and approach a community diagnosis by asking, 'What sort of a common medical problems do you have in this community?' You interacted with the community right from the word 'go,'" she said. "I have to be honest. It was intimidating. But now I have no problem walking into any community or into any county office and express myself and really talk about what I want to do," she said. "And I

Facing, Ambulances come and go from the front entrance of the Riley Mother and Baby Hospital, where Julia Songok has worked as a pediatrician since the opening day in 2009. She was then and remains the department head of the Newborn Unit at the MTRH. The "mother/baby" hospital is named after the world-famous Riley Hospital for Children in Indianapolis where Julia completed a five-month residency fellowship before returning to AMPATH in 2000. Julia thinks of herself as a Kenyan child of AMPATH.

can also listen, because we learned medicine in a collaborative way."

Julia appreciates the difference that one person, such as Mengech, can make. At the start of the medical school, he and his IU partners created a curriculum that emphasized collaboration among the students solving the real-life problems they were seeing on the hospital wards and in clinics out in the villages. "I think it takes a courageous person to think through something like that. Today, we don't struggle to think about the patient and the family and the community," she said. "It is not until you interact with someone who has been trained a different system and who lives in a different environment that you realize, 'Oh, it's actually not the norm. What we have is special.'"

Julia completed her medical degree in 1999 and began working at MTRH. When I spoke with her in May 2019, she seemed quite comfortable in the office given to the head of child health and pediatrics in what is now the Moi University School of Medicine. She reflected on many mentors who had encouraged her.

She spoke first of Mengech and the innovations he provided to medical education. She then mentioned James Lemons, the IU pediatrics professor who was instrumental in building the Riley Mother Baby Hospital, where Julia does her clinical rounds. "There were so many discussions, so many tutorials with Prof Lemons and the great teachers: Joe Mamlin, Constance Tenge, David Matthews, Samwel Ayaya, Fabian Esamai, Bob Einterz, and so many." These Kenyan and American doctors were learning about teaching in a new way, and their students sensed the excitement and were encouraged.

She explained how these professors made her feel appreciated. "We had these amazing mentors that we looked up to for so much, not just for academics but just professionalism. We wanted to be that kind of doctor,"

she said. "I think the feeling of support was like literally standing on the shoulders of giants. It's Professor Mamlin. It's Professor Kimaiyo. It's Dr. Adrian Gardner. Oh, and it's Prof Einterz. I stayed at his house when I was a medical student," she continued. "So, when people talk about giants, it sounds imaginary, and it sounds like it's in the movies. But the honest truth about AMPATH is that these have been true giants. Despite the heavy workload that AMPATH demanded, they were still good clinicians. They still are, and they are still our mentors."

Toward the end of her medical school education in 1997, Julia got to travel to Indianapolis to spend eight weeks at the Riley Hospital for Children with her teacher James Lemons. "And it was it was such an eye opener," she said. "There was so much to learn, but there was also so much culture shock. . . . There were so many differences in terms of the kind of disease pattern, the gravity of the pathology that we saw amongst the patients, but also in the medical culture. There was so much mentorship in Indianapolis."

Julia completed her degree, did her internship at MTRH, and then, after working for three years in pediatrics in Eldoret, started her residency, which included a return to Indiana for a five-month resident fellowship. "Unlike the earlier time, when I was that medical student and everything was a shock, going back as a resident I was actually able to identify certain things that would be practical back in Kenya," she said. "I came home with new ideas."

Upon her return to Kenya, she was required to spend time working for AMPATH, where the mentoring continued. Every Tuesday she would meet with Winstone Nyandiko, head of research. "I was taking time to understand the approaches of treatment, to understand decision making, and just ask questions and be asked questions. And that was also something that allowed me to understand AMPATH in depth."

In 2007, AMPATH received the first funding for primary healthcare, and Julia was added to the team the next year. AMPATH's HIV program had good systems in place by then. The public healthcare officials working out of the MTRH looked at the system components built to combat HIV and basically copied them into the public healthcare system. They worked closely with people in the villages to create systems that used community healthcare workers and community extension workers so they could really understand both the common conditions as well as the uniqueness of the illnesses within the region. "That really allowed me to understand not just AMPATH but also understand the communities and how the healthcare system can help," she said.

It was increasingly clear to Julia that the academic model that addressed the HIV crisis so effectively could be put to work to address primary healthcare issues ranging from childbirth to chronic diseases. Community-based groups like GISHE, MamaToto, and community health volunteers could also be used to deliver all manner of healthcare. "I really managed to piece together my understanding of the community-based educational services that we worked with during my entire six years of medical student training," she said. "Every year there was a community component where you actually go to a small rural area and spend up to six weeks just making a community diagnosis."

Julia said this allowed her to connect her experience working in village clinics as a medical school with what she now understands as AMPATH's theories about community collaboration. The academic model for medical education—providing care directly at the village level— had all along been a program fostering public health.

The ubiquity of AMPATH's approach and method is easy to see in Julia's career as she has moved from student to intern to resident to attending and now department head. "You know, the beauty of AMPATH is that whether you are at MTRH or Moi University, you are under the same umbrella," she said. "Even if we change employers within, there is still relevance to the work of AMPATH, and you can still be part of that team."

"Working with North Americans has really opened up my mind," she said. "For the longest time, I've watched Dr. Laura Ruhl. I met her when she was a medical student visiting here. She came back as a resident, and we met again, and now we work together on the primary healthcare grant that has come through USAID."

Julia and Laura are two of many women who were advantaged by a system that not only integrated experiential learning into the curriculum but also encouraged women to aspire to the highest levels of achievement in what remains a male-dominant profession. Julia sees clearly how empowering the hands-on approach championed by Mengech and the folks at IU has been. "The ability to not just provide care but also understand how to write grants, to access resources, to be able to implement innovative ideas that we have had . . . to me that was really amazing because without that collaboration, I would not have had that chance. It's been a really great journey," she said.

These days Julia harnesses these skills in an effort to bring universal healthcare to Kenya through the population health model headed by her friends Laura Ruhl and Jeremiah Laktabai. "It is the embracing of all the different community challenges that defines universal health, and it's the national insurance system that allows patients to access the care they need. When you design something that is really good, and patients can access and utilize the resources, then we can talk of a whole process that is truly

Facing, There is a teaching room just two floors below the office Paul Ayuo occupied as principal of the Moi University College of Health Sciences in 2019. Ayuo prefers being in the classroom because he can be among his students. He joined the Moi University School of Medicine in 1992 as a lecturer just as it was getting started. He rose to become a professor of medicine and then dean of the school. Even while serving as the college's top administrator, he regularly led the AMPATH Training Institute.

sustainable," she said. "All these teams that are working on different things in terms of sustainability and access, they have all our support because we know that every single Kenyan, at some point, will have to be on board and be taken care of in the context of population health."

I mentioned that it seemed to me that the students Mengech and Joe and Bob had taught way back in the 1990s were now taking over. She replied, "Yes, we are taking over, but the truth is that the relationships and the collaboration are key even in the takeover. It may be that Kenyans will play a bigger role, maybe, but we still need the collaboration. We still need the consortium. The roles may change a little bit over time, but the sure truth is we need them. I need them still."

Paul Ayuo

The Moi University College of Health Sciences' four-story, poured-concrete building sits just across Nandi Road from the equally tall but gleaming blue, glass-clad Chandaria Centre building. As principal of the college, Professor Paul Ayuo shared AMPATH Executive Board leadership with Wilson Aruasa, the CEO of the MTRH. Their window views of each other's operations is perhaps symbolic of their relationship. When I met with Ayuo in 2019, he and Aruasa together headed a unique partnership that accounts for the success of the larger collaboration with the North American consortium.

Ayuo greeted me from his executive desk and offered me a glass of fresh mango juice. His graduation gown hung in the far corner of the room. It was clear from the start of the interview that Ayuo is a teacher. He was happy to school me.

"I joined what was then called the Faculty of Health Sciences in 1992," he said and then mentioned that he was one of only two Kenyan physicians on the faculty.

The medical school was just four years old, and the first students had matriculated only two years earlier. Indiana University had been partnering with the new school since the beginning, and everyone was eager to graduate the first class of medical students.

"Professor Joe Mamlin of IU was the long-term resident about then. We rounded with him on all of the medical wards and taught the students what we knew," he recalled. "Apart from being an excellent teacher, even to myself, Joe had a way of befriending his patients. Sometimes he would bring them gifts, but most significantly, he brought medicines that were missing from the hospital stock."

Joe and Sarah Ellen Mamlin were living full time in Eldoret while Joe was the field director for the IU-Kenya Partnership. Bob and Lea Anne Einterz had preceded them, and the plan was to keep an American doctor in Eldoret full time as Moi's new medical school matured. The Mamlins returned home in 1993 and Joe became chief of medicine at IU's Wishard Memorial Hospital in Indianapolis. Ayuo, naturally, stayed in Eldoret and was head of the Moi University School of Medicine by 2000 when the Mamlins returned to Eldoret following Joe's retirement.

The Mamlins found that their friend Ayuo was in the midst of an AIDS crisis that was driving the staff to despair. Ayuo was happy to see his old colleague again and have him rejoin his department, but he was struggling to teach students about an illness for which there was no cure or ready therapy. Within a year, however, he and Joe were *treating* AIDS patients instead of simply assisting them as they died on hospital wards where the two old friends had together once taught young students that anything was possible.

Ayuo recalled the difficulty of those early days of the epidemic. "Sometimes we had a very limited amount of drugs. We would sit as a committee and say, 'All right,

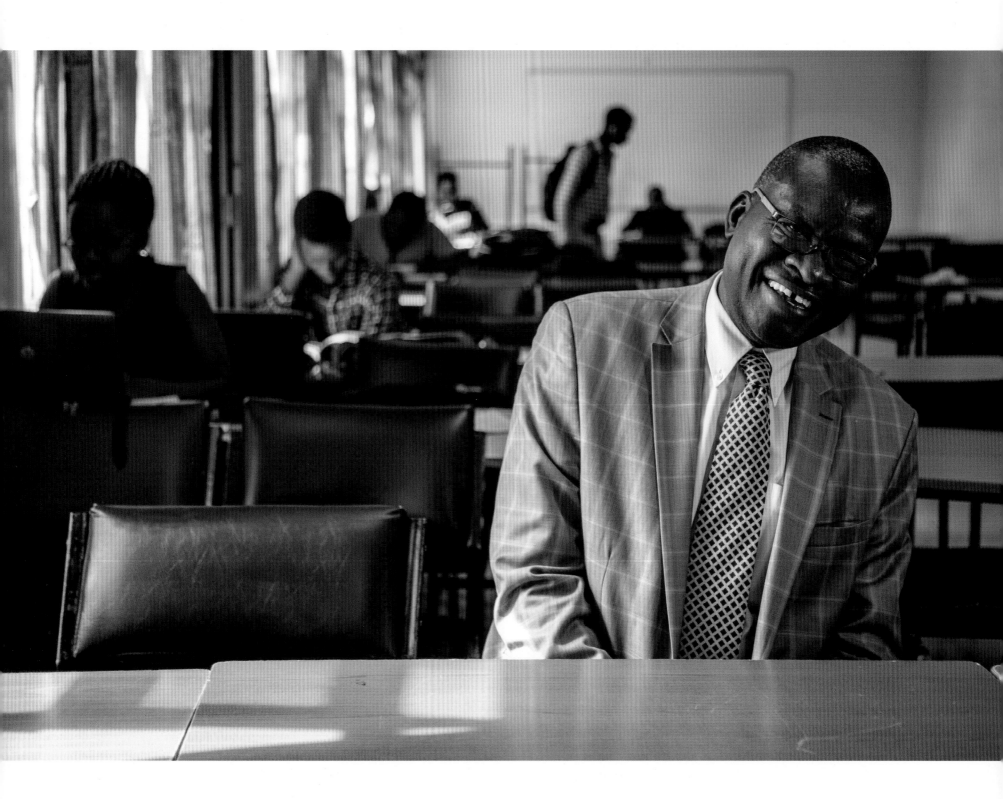

identify five patients from the people you are looking over,' knowing that we would be left without drugs for the others." There were trying times when dozens died of AIDS on the wards every week. The modest grants Joe and Bob had secured in the earliest days of the treatment phase of the epidemic provided drugs to treat many, but not all.

About that same time, Sylvester Kimaiyo, a graduate of the University of Nairobi's medical school whom Ayuo had only recently hired onto the faculty, left for Indiana, where he spent a year training in HIV care. "Professor Kimaiyo came back to us in 2002 and took direction over the whole HIV care program," Ayuo recalled. While Kimaiyo was away, HIV care had been transformed by the drugs donated by folks in Indiana, and there was hope that the epidemic could be managed if only more funding could be had.

Ayuo soon joined with Kimaiyo and his IU partners on a grant proposal submitted to USAID by a newly created organization they called AMPATH: The Academic Model for the Prevention and Treatment of HIV/AIDS. Ayuo explained that "AMPATH was an acronym coined as a vehicle to apply for federal funding in 2004 from PEP-FAR," which was yet another acronym for the President's Emergency Plan for AIDS Relief, the multimillion-dollar program generally credited with stemming the tide of the epidemic in Africa. "When PEPFAR came, I think most people who required treatment got the treatment they needed," he recalled.

Throughout the crisis years, Ayuo and the Moi medical program continued training doctors. The old professor spoke with great gratitude about the Mwangaza scholarships that sustained many of those early clinical trainees and how needy students continue to benefit from the program. The Mwangaza scholarships were first awarded to Moi students in 2000. Before that, many Kenyan students skipped meals to pay tuition and fees. Ten years later, nearly 30 percent of students pursuing medical degrees at Moi were receiving scholarships, and many more were supported by work-study funded by AMPATH. And a decade later still, eighteen to twenty Moi medical students were participating in educational exchanges at one of the North American AMPATH institutions every year. More than four hundred medical students from Moi have spent time training in Indianapolis or at another consortium university since 1995 (Turissini et al. 2020). Students are regularly amazed by the state-of-the-art facilities and the relative wealth of the cities they temporarily call home. They return to Eldoret with new ideas and enthusiasm.

In true partnership, Ayuo and his Moi colleagues host a regular stream of North American medical students in the MTRH and their Moi classrooms. Matt Turissini and his colleagues, including Ayuo, concluded that 1,871 North American medical and pharmacy students have studied at Moi since the start of the partnership. For about half of each student's two-month stay they live in the Moi student dormitory/hostel located just across Nandi Road from the hospital and the other half at the IU House. The hostel rooms are much smaller than the *wazungu* are used to, but the hostel experience provides a fertile seedbed for friendships with Moi students that last a lifetime.

The unique opportunity "allows for a more immersive experience and facilitates the development of counterpart relationships that are the bedrock of the program" (6). While in Eldoret, the forty to fifty students in a typical year rise before the sun, do daily rounds with the MTRH staff and their Kenyan colleagues, and then study in their shared hostel rooms all evening. According to Turissini and colleagues, "AMPATH exchange participants were more likely to provide care to underserved populations, consider cost in clinical-care decisions, and be involved in public health policy and advocacy" (6).

"When our Moi students go to the US, they are basically 'economically deprived' compared to the US students who come here and pay their own way. Our students cannot pay there. The American side of the collaboration gets them air tickets, they get hosted, and they live with families for the six weeks they are in the US," Ayuo said. "It's a beautiful experience."

He spoke appreciatively of the other benefits Moi has derived from the partnership over the years. "Some people have gone back for residency in the US and are now successful people working at MTRH. There's been a lot of benefits. We have new buildings here now," he said. "We used to have one dilapidated theater [operating room] in MTRH. Then in 2000 an IU surgeon named Dave Matthews mobilized a funds drive through his Presbyterian church in Indianapolis, and they built four theaters. It was the biggest thing to happen to surgery in the hospital."

Ayuo himself occasionally visits the US to raise funds for AMAPTH and recalled one visit with a donor in Rhode Island. He said, "Bob Einterz and I were going around visiting our partners and trying to see how we could raise funds. We go to this meeting at a private club and the memorable thing about it is that Jane Carter, the woman we were asking for funds [a Brown University physician who mentored Adrian Gardner], she was the first woman to be admitted into that club. Before that, it was a club of men only. That was the first time we had heard of a thing like that in America!"

"We can talk about the lives impacted by these donations in Kenya, millions of people affected and infected with HIV plus their relatives," he continued. "But there is also something that is not normally mentioned, and this is on a personal level. When people come here, we make friends. I've known many people who have gone abroad and were supported on a personal level and not just a program level. There are so many things from personal experiences to institutional experiences that we have accrued from this collaboration."

According to Ayuo, "The thing is that when you collaborate, you must look at each other as equal partners. It's not a master/servant kind of relationship. This is the strongest point about our collaboration with North America. We work as a team and as equal partners always."

He talked about the difference between trainings and partnerships. "Most of the North-South partnerships are mostly trainings. The North comes and says, 'We've got this research project we want to do.' They do it and then they take off." He said that Moi's relationship with the folks at AMPATH has always been different. "We had a common interest that was unique in the sense that the things we were feeling were also being felt by those people from Indiana. It's why we created the term Leading with Care because we all believed that, first, you must do care. We needed to be able to teach, and we needed to be able to do some research. But the care always comes first. Then teaching follows," he said. "And finally, research informs the care. It's kind of a cycle that we all believed in from the start."

"The idea was always of being equal partners and having counterparts," he said. "If you have a committee, for example, there's a Kenyan and a North American as cochairs. I think it's that common understanding of the problem that we need to solve and an agreed-upon method that has kept this going. And, of course, it's been the generous donations resulting from our grant proposals from the agencies that fund us. They believe in us, and that's extremely motivating."

I asked Ayuo how this philosophy of equality and focus on care influences the students who study under him at the college and then become members of the staff. He replied, "At first I would say it is the outcome of one's work that gives motivation. It is quite motivating to work

The revolving fund pharmacy (RFP) on the ground floor of the AMPATH Centre seems a bit redundant since the Ministry of Health pharmacy is just down the hall and is three times as large. Sonak Pastakia, the Purdue Kenya Program team leader in Eldoret since 2009, will tell you it provides backup supplies of crucial medications in the event that pharmacies in government health facilities are depleted. Sonak, a professor of pharmacy practice, helped create the RFP initiative in 2013. They now operate in nearly twenty AMPATH clinics.

for AMPATH, to be associated with its success and also see the fruits of our work. People are surely getting better because these staff work hard. It's not like before when people were dying of AIDS. A second reason is the leadership. People know the leadership is working for them and that education is important."

I also ask about his ability to keep faculty physicians at Moi, especially given the fact that he encourages them to go to the US for training. "Some people do emigrate, but generally, I think Kenyans are not the emigrating type, if you compare them to other countries in East or West Africa. Kenyans tend to stay in their jobs much longer," he explained. "But as I said before, it is the end product of your work that makes for high job satisfaction. Where you have high job satisfaction, you have people who are likely to stay longer," he asserted. "The other thing is that most of us here are employed by the MTRH or by Moi University. We are here working to better our country, and we gain satisfaction working with the North Americans in AMPATH. But for most of our employees outside Eldoret—the outreach and the health centers in the field—I think the main thing is the satisfaction of helping." I learned a lot from my time with the professor.

Sonak Pastakia

Professor Sonak Pastakia's house was one of four houses in a compound of buildings just up the lane from the IU House owned by Mr. Noah Ngeny, an Olympic gold medalist in the 1,500 meters and world record holder in the 1,000-meter race. My wife and I lived in one of the smaller houses that surrounded Noah's big house, as did Sonak. For five months, I sat in my home study overlooking the parking lot and watched Sonak and Professor Rakhi Karwa, his wife and fellow pharmacy professor, as they loaded and unloaded their two preschool-aged daughters

in and out of the family car. It was a window onto a happy family. Their Indian parents had migrated to Philadelphia and Cleveland in search of a better life a generation earlier, and now they were living in a small city in rural Africa where poverty is high and economic development is too low. Like their immigrant parents, they were in search of a better life—for themselves and for others.

I met with Sonak in his family's dining room at a table littered with his daughters' school papers. He started with a story about one of his pharmacy students: Mr. Benson Kiragu. "I marvel at the extremes of resilience among this population. People you saw on the street one day and never imagined they could do anything are now the people changing things across the country," he said, talking about Benson.

"Benson was a street youth, and he kind of ties together all the different pieces of AMPATH," he continued. The Mamlins used to visit a day center for children who had fled their villages to find refuge living on the streets of Eldoret. That was 2002—a time when AIDS was creating orphans across sub-Saharan Africa. "Joe Mamlin would provide weekly checkups for all these kids who were living on the streets. Benson had eye problems, so even after the Mamlins got him into a school, he struggled to see the chalkboard. Plus, he had asthma that was frequently exacerbated by the dust and cold weather he had been exposed to from living on the street for so long," he said. "Joe and Sarah Ellen effectively adopted him and permanently changed the course of Benson's life."

At the request of IU leadership, Purdue University's Department of Pharmacy Practice joined the new AMPATH Consortium in 2003 to help develop supply-chain solutions. Professor Julie Everett headed the effort in Eldoret. "Benson became the de facto liaison to the Purdue students that she would bring over. He would show them the town, get them into the culture of Kenya, and

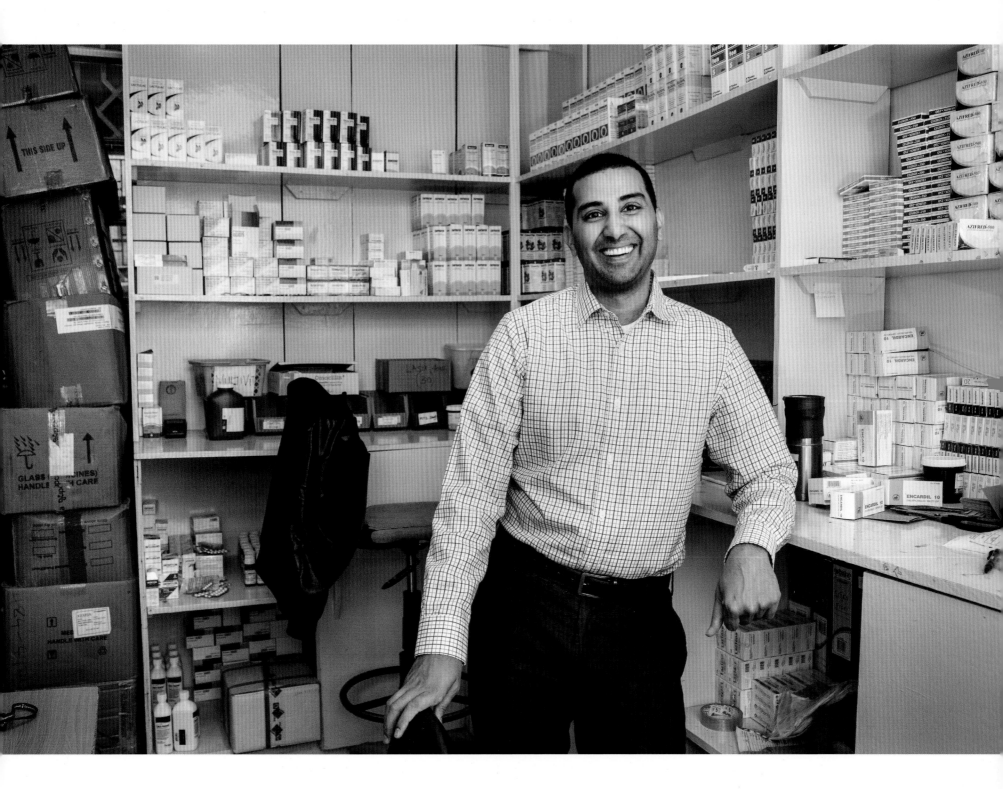

help them with the practical matters of living in Kenya," Sonak explained. "Benson would say to Julie, 'I want to be like you someday. I want to be a pharmacist.'" Sadly, Julie died in 2006, and Sonak was hired the following year to lead Purdue's presence in Kenya. Before long he had Benson working in the AMPATH pharmacy, repackaging medicines and such, and was encouraging him to pursue whatever career path he wanted. Because of his prior commitment to Julie and his desire to follow in her footsteps, Benson was adamant about becoming a pharmacist after high school. Despite having a host of sponsors willing to financially support him, admittance to Kenyan universities required a B average, and Benson had a C+.

Sonak continued, "So, Benson being who Benson is, he figured out he could get into a university in the Philippines and study for a pharmacy degree there. We sponsored him to go there, he returned to Eldoret with a degree, and joined the team I work with now."

"This is street kid who'd had three or four corneal transplants, has eye problems that very few could ever even imagine, and is currently blind in one eye. He highlights the resilience of people here. All he needed was a couple points of support in order for him to reach his goal of being a pharmacist and giving back to his community," he said.

Benson has benefitted from the long-term commitment that Sonak, early in his training, realized was necessary for lasting change. "While I was a pharmacy resident, I was very excited about getting experience outside the United States and thought I knew more than I did. In 2004, I joined a group that went to Kenya every year for four-week visits. The goal was to set up primary care in Kisumu, which was then a hot spot for HIV in Kenya," he recalled. Kisumu is just seventy-five miles southwest of Eldoret but was not quite yet in the AMPATH catchment area.

"We set up makeshift, free clinics in government facilities," he said. "We would give out free medicines. At first, I thought, 'This is great. We are helping so many people.' But more and more patients were coming with obvious signs of HIV and late-stage AIDS, and the best we did was to diagnose them and send them to facilities we knew did not have the necessary drugs to treat them. And it was not just AIDS patients that came for our free care. We had people showing up with gaping wounds, hypertension, malaria, and other conditions we simply could not treat effectively with episodic care we delivered based on our convenience."

According to Sonak, "This whole group of mostly white folks arrived every year at the same time of the year. People waited to get the free care from these 'white saviors.' Over time, I felt myself getting more and more jaded and more and more frustrated. As healthcare providers, we knew what we were seeing. But the best we could do for these patients was to give them a temporary solution before packing our bags and going."

"We wanted to feel like saviors without considering the patients' real needs. The whole notion of establishing primary care for just one month out of every year was ridiculous. No one would suggest that would be possible in a resource-rich setting like America, but for some reason, we thought it was good for Africa," he said.

"On the thirty-six-hour flight back home, I was so ridden with guilt that I basically changed my whole career plan. What could I do to atone for this? How could I be part of something that was truly responsive? The patients in Kisumu had done their part. . . . We came abysmally short of meeting their expectations," he conceded.

Upon return to the US, Sonak completed an infectious diseases residency at the University of North Carolina Hospital, which was one of the main centers providing HIV care for underserved populations at the time. He then went looking for a job at a program that could deliver care and training on a long-term basis. It had to immerse students in effective patient care, promote evidence-based care, and also generate useful research. He couldn't find such a place until one of the people he had interviewed with sent him a posting from Purdue. He said, "I emailed Purdue in 2006, interviewed, fell in love with the program, and said I'd go anywhere in the world that enabled me to have a more useful role in helping patients than what I previously imagined doing in America." They sent him back to Kenya.

"Upon joining AMPATH, I rounded with Joe Mamlin to start off. We probably had five or six thousand HIV-positive patients at the time in our outpatient care program in western Kenya," he said. "And I was completely overwhelmed."

"I was used to seeing HIV patients in a US context. Joe was used to seeing HIV patients in a Kenyan context. Every patient we saw on the wards would've warranted intensive care in the US, but here patients were two to a bed. They were getting drugs for HIV, but many were not getting the care they needed for the other equally life-threatening conditions they had, even though that treatment was readily available and had been prescribed," he said. "All they needed was somebody to make sure they were getting their drugs."

Purdue pharmacy students were coming to Eldoret and training in multiple aspects of the Kenyan healthcare system for eight weeks but then taking their new knowledge back to Indiana. Sonak was frustrated by what seemed too similar to the program in Kisumu years earlier.

"I had been working with technicians in the main pharmacy at MTRH and noticed there were a bunch of Kenyan . . . interns from the University of Nairobi who had completed their degrees and had been posted to MTRH for their rotations. They told me that there wasn't

any work for them. I said, 'No, no, no, no, no. Come with me. We've got lots of work.' They were sitting in the midst of a healthcare crisis, but no one was taking the time to see how they could be part of the response," he said.

"Our programs then shifted from being US-student focused to Kenyan-student focused. We incorporated these Kenyan pharmacists into our training system—same as we were doing with the Purdue students. The Kenyans had never seen clinical pharmacy before. They could recite complete textbooks, protocols, and guidelines, but when it came to applying their knowledge, there had never been anyone who could train them to really apply their knowledge to patient care in a clinical setting," he recalled.

The University of Nairobi had the only accredited pharmacy program in Kenya when Sonak joined AMPATH. Like so much of the country's higher education, instruction was almost exclusively theoretical. Students learned from books and lectures, not from hands-on practical experience in hospitals and clinics (Ogaji et al. 2016).

"For our American students, clinical training was the foundation of their education. Their knowledge was grounded in experience and complemented by the didactics. When I set the Kenyans to do this, I was blown away. The Kenyans were able to apply their substantial theoretical knowledge in a human context where it wasn't just one illness, but HIV, high blood pressure, meningitis, and other things. They'd never been trained to apply their textbook knowledge to practical things."

He concluded, "After just a couple of weeks, the Kenyan students were surpassing all of the expectations I had for them. From that point forward, our model was always integrated—American students training side by side with Kenyan students."

The lessons for the Purdue students were similarly extraordinary. After a relatively brief meeting where incoming Americans talked with their Kenyan counterparts, Sonak said, "all the false notions that one side had about the other went out the window. By the end of the meeting, the Purdue students' worldview had changed. They recognize the strength of the Kenyans' education, and old notions of African helplessness went out the window too. 'Holy moly, I need to learn from these folks because they know what they are talking about,' they would say."

The North Americans had more advanced knowledge and experience with chronic diseases like hypertension and diabetes, whereas the Kenyan students had greater knowledge of gastroenteritis, HIV, tuberculosis (TB), and things they see a lot more often. The students realized they had much to learn from each other. "It was a synergistic combination," he said.

"Today we have transitioned all the pharmacists who used to be just behind the window dispensing drugs to a completely different job role where they are now clinical pharmacists working on the wards, doing direct patient care. We offer a postgraduate diploma in pharmacy as well as a master's degree in clinical pharmacy, and we train interns from all of the schools of pharmacy in Kenya. We have created a model for clinical pharmacy that can be replicated across the country," he said.

"When you go out to the community hospitals, you'll find clinical pharmacists there as well. We now have seventy-six revolving-fund pharmacies that serve as a backup supply chain to the Ministry of Health. Many are staffed by the very pharmacists we have trained," he said.

The revolving-fund pharmacy model provides high-quality medications consistently to patients by using revenues generated from the sale of medications to sustainably resupply medications. The system works as a complement to the government supply of medicines that are subsidized but frequently out of stock.

"Everything comes full circle. We were out to set up care infrastructure, add students on to it, and do research. We have enough fully trained pharmacists now who lead the research while I ride their coattails," he said. It is the circle that Sonak set out to complete during his long airplane ride home from Kisumu more than fifteen years earlier. I asked him why he and his colleagues had been able to accomplish this.

"It's about people. It's about somebody having a vision and saying, 'We are going to do this the right way despite all of the people who tell us it can't be done.' It's people who say yes when everyone else says no," he replied. "When the global medical community was saying that a generation of Africans would have to die of AIDS because prevention was the only way to address the epidemic, a visionary like Joe Mamlin said, 'We can treat them.' He said that because he had built relationships with the people in Eldoret who were living in the midst of an epidemic. They did it together."

"Credit goes to IU for taking the chance on a program like the IU-Kenya Partnership, and credit goes to Purdue for joining AMPATH. The vast majority of universities were unwilling to take on a project like that. It was a low-reward program in the early days when things were uncertain and risks were high," Sonak concluded. "But the potential for rewards in the long term was exponential. The rewards AMPATH is reaping for faculty like me and most importantly for the hundreds of thousands of patients AMPATH serves today are great."

Adrian Gardner

The Consortium Space in the Chandaria Centre is a huge room of modular desks, cardboard boxes, and stacks and stacks of file folders. For most of the North Americans working with AMPATH, it is their office in Eldoret where

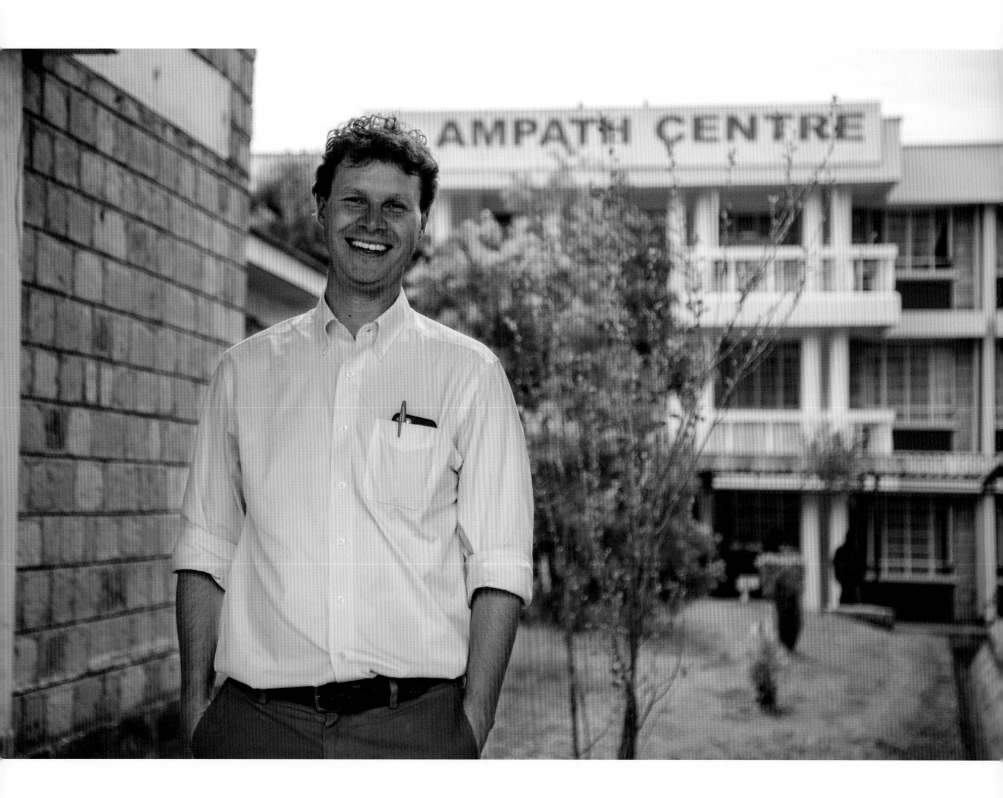

they can work on their laptops, read reports, or maybe meet with colleagues over burritos ordered for delivery from Sizzlers Cafe on Thursdays. Everywhere else in the massive healthcare system that serves western Kenya, the foreigners are always in Kenyan spaces. They are welcome there and made to feel at home, but every ward, every clinic, every dispensary is someone else's place. The Consortium Space is for the *wazungu*.

In the corner of the space is a small office with a sign on the door that says AMPATH Field Director. It is nearly always open. Behind a desk handed down from some system administrator years ago when the building was new is Dr. Adrian Gardner, who sits on a chair with a broken wheel and a tear in the vinyl covering the right armrest. At the time I met with him in 2019, he had been executive field director of the AMPATH Consortium for eight years, but his engagement with Kenyans went back much further.

He recalled,

I got here the first time about a week before 9/11, 2001. It was a unique time. There was no one else coming from North America after the attack in New York. There were four or five of us medical students and residents here, and Joe and Sarah Ellen. It was a weird time to be away from home. We weren't getting 24-7 news coverage. The only TV was in the hospital cafeteria. We were getting some updates, but it was not the immediate coverage that everybody was experiencing back home. I had friends in Manhattan and was concerned about them.

Having experienced the bombing of the US embassy in Nairobi in 1988, many Kenyans could and did relate to the loss of life and feeling of insecurity. They comforted their American friends as best they could.

At that time, Adrian was a fourth-year medical student at Brown University in Rhode Island. "There was no

AMPATH yet. Joe had only returned a year earlier and was probably just conceiving of it," he said. There was AIDS, however.

In 2001, the United Nations estimated that 28 million people on the continent were infected with HIV, 2.3 million Africans had died from AIDS-related illnesses, and 3.4 million were newly infected. The wards of MTRH were crowded with AIDS patients. Joe had been back in Kenya as field director for just one year. He and his Kenyan colleagues were treating a small number of HIV patients with donated drugs and small grants of money from friends back in Indiana.

"My time in Eldoret was a life-changing experience. It changed my career path," Adrian said. "I had wanted to be a maternal-fetal medicine doctor. When I came here and saw the enormous burden of medical illness, I thought, 'Maybe women can deliver babies without my help?' Of course, that was naive because there were huge needs in obstetrics and maternal-child care as well. What I appreciated was this emerging epidemic that demanded response."

It was not the first time Adrian had run into HIV. His father had worked for the Merck pharmaceutical company in Pennsylvania while Adrian was in high school. "I did a summer internship at Merck. They were doing clinical trials and developing the first protease inhibitor for HIV. It was a completely new class of drugs for HIV," he recalled. "And so, I guess that was my first connection to HIV."

His second connection was as a freshman at Brown University. "I worked as a volunteer in an AIDS orphanage in Providence. We would just go down and play with these kids for four hours a week," he said. "I hadn't really thought of those things as connected, but I guess in some ways, I have been gravitating toward this work for a long time."

After those two months as a student at Moi in 2001, Adrian returned to Rhode Island and spent the rest of his fourth year of medical school in a longitudinal TB clinic in Providence with Dr. Jane Carter, then the TB/HIV technical consultant for AMPATH and a wonderful mentor. These experiences in Kenya and Providence inspired Adrian to pursue global health training by pursuing a Master of Public Health degree at Harvard.

"It was a wonderful time to process my experience in Kenya," he said. "The Harvard School of Public Health attracted amazing people. One of my classmates was the head of Médecins Sans Frontières in China, for example." Adrian was so engaged in all the talk of international development that he spent his only three-week break visiting Eldoret, just to see how things were going. As Adrian talked, he shifted his weight forward toward the desk and got a jolt as the broken chair collapsed on the leg missing its wheel. The man with two Ivy league graduate degrees didn't even break sentence. Chairs were not important. Service was.

By 2006 he had finished his residency at Beth Israel Deaconess Medical Center in Boston and was back in Eldoret full time as the medicine team leader for AMPATH. Since the start of the partnership between IU and Moi, an IU doctor was resident for a year in Eldoret to practice medicine, teach at Moi University, and oversee Indiana students and residents. Bob Einterz had been the first team leader in 1990. Charlie Kelley had taken a turn, as had Joe Mamlin, David Van Reken, Gregory Gramelspacher, John Sidle, and others. Adrian was the fourteenth. He followed his friend Dr. Rajesh Vedanthan as medicine team leader and joined Dr. Jason Woodward, the pediatric team leader that year.

"I was seeing patients in MTRH and going out to the AMPATH clinic in Turbo every Tuesday," Adrian said. "I was doing the work I had trained for, and it really cemented my commitment to AMPATH." However, shortly after arriving for what he had imagined would be a one-year stint as leader, he applied for an infectious diseases fellowship in Boston, where he had done his residency and had met an intensive care unit nurse. "I told the fellowship director, 'I would really like to spend another year here in Kenya. Could I delay my fellowship?' And basically, after some discussion, she said no."

So Adrian returned to New England once again, completed his fellowship, and then married Ms. Jessica Geibel, the nurse he had returned home to be with. And he began wondering whether he could ever persuade his new wife to move to rural Kenya and raise a family there. "I was thinking about AMPATH the whole time I was in Boston. I spent a lot of time in clinical HIV—four days a week—which is much more time than most people would do as part of the fellowship." One of the clinics was in a public hospital that served "the down and out." It was a lot of work, but Adrian had Jess's support and encouragement.

"When the opportunity to apply for the AMPATH field director job came up in 2011, it was a no-brainer for me," he said. "But it was far more challenging for Jess. She had just finished anesthesia school and was pregnant. She had only been to Africa once, to visit me, so it was a big deal for her to leave family and a good job and move to rural Kenya at five months into her pregnancy."

"Obviously, we've committed ourselves to being here now," he said. "This is our home. We have two daughters now, and they are growing up in this wonderful community." I mentioned that I'd seen Jess and their oldest daughter at the Imani Workshop a few days earlier. The workshop began fifteen years ago as a place where HIV-positive people could learn craft-making skills and earn a living. It has a shop that offers their products. Adrian said, "And do you know what she bought? She bought earrings for her two nannies. She told me this morning that she bought them the same pair because she didn't want one to feel jealous of the other. She's just a very thoughtful individual, very caring."

Adrian admits that life in Eldoret differs considerably from the life he and Jess might have had in Boston. He tells me about one of the students he went to school with who now has a practice in Manhattan and pays $1,000 a week for a nanny to care for his children. "We have help with the girls here too, and it's nice. It allows you time to do what you want to do, which is a real privilege. But it also allows you to commit yourself more to work."

As executive field director, Adrian's work is increasingly managing relationships with partners. AMPATH itself is a consortium of more than a dozen university partners all working with Moi University and MTRH to produce innovations in healthcare. That work, in turn, is sustained by dozens of additional partners: US and Kenyan government agencies, private foundations, international funders, and pharmaceutical companies.

When I had asked Adrian's Kenyan counterpart, AMPATH Plus chief of party Sylvester Kimaiyo, why foreign donors and partners trust that the money they give won't be lost to corruption, he told me the key was the Research and Sponsored Projects Office. He explained that RSPO provided the fiscal accounting required by various funders, especially USAID, and that it was the reason AMPATH could operate so efficiently in a country plagued with corruption. I still didn't understand how it worked, so I asked Adrian.

"RSPO is not a legal entity. It's this sort of nebulous thing in the balance of AMPATH as a collaboration of institutions. It's the place where AMPATH becomes the most real in my mind," he said. "Our people often work for more than one organization. Some more work for AMPATH and MTRH, some work for AMPATH and for Moi University, some work for AMPATH and a consortium university,

and others are contract staff hired by one of the projects to run grants and extramural funding for these institutions." RSPO is "an essential piece of the infrastructure that has been really necessary to make it all work," he explained.

Adrian told me about how, in 2012, USAID awarded the multimillion-dollar PEPFAR grant to MTRH as the "prime" rather than to IU. The "prime" is the institution responsible for managing the project and accounting for the money spent to do so. He said, "A lot of eyes in Washington were looking down on this and saying, 'You AID guys are crazy to send this money to a Kenyan public institution with a history of corruption.' The reality on the ground was different, but it was hard to explain that to people, and it's still hard to explain that to some of our prospective donors."

A few years later, the World Bank was about to fund a substantial project. Adrian described the contact person as saying, "So, we are going to grant the money to MTRH or Moi University as the legal entity, but you're telling me the money is going to be managed outside of those institutions? It's not going to go into the government's account? How is that going to work? I look at the audit report for many public institutions in Kenya, and it says they're insolvent. They're not paying their salaries. How can I possibly put money in this institution?" And Adrian told him, "Well, it's not actually going there. Your money is going to our RSPO. These guys have passed six years of audits by Deloitte-level accountants, and they manage up to NIH and USAID standards. They pass the tests" but are still accountable to the heads of MTRH and Moi University.

The RSPO was AMPATH's method for providing the financial assurance needed to get grants flowing directly into Eldoret. It grew out of the financial accounting system the IU House had set up back in the 1990s to handle small donations to support the partnership. Since 2003, RSPO has been headed by Mr. Robert Rono. He and

Ms. Christine Chuani (who is now at MTRH doing similar work) were tapped by Joe Mamlin, who showed them how the IU House system was run. According to Rono, "The RSPO was set up to be 'semi-autonomous' from the MTRH and Moi University, which are very bureaucratic. We work within regulations of the donors: mostly with foreign funders, though a few have grants from Kenyan government." From an office of two, they have grown to over one hundred employees overseeing awards averaging $30 million annually. One of his teams manages the USAID/PEPFAR award, and another team manages all other grants. Rono concluded, "We manage from preaward, application submission, budget management, reporting on the finances to the funder, to final reporting."

Adrian explained that international funders had previously insisted a Western institution like IU be the prime recipient but "they are now saying, 'OK, we are reaching out to Moi University or MTRH, and we are going to send the money to them, and the project is going to be run by Kenyans.' They don't see a need for a subcontract to Indiana University" because the RSPO manages it so efficiently. "I think this is good, but it requires a decision for us about the nature of our partnership. It's a new era."

The new era is essentially the same one described in the population health plan headed by Laktabai and Ruhl. AMPATH Consortium members will increasingly work with MTRH and Moi University on projects they manage rather than the other way around. Experts from North America will contribute to funded projects, and they may in some cases even be principal investigators, but the grants will be administered by Kenyans in the RSPO and, more often than not, will be led by Kenyans in MTRH and Moi. There will be no support going through IU or any other consortium member.

"I think it creates new challenges, but not insurmountable ones," Adrian said. "The question is how well will relationships be maintained between the funders and the project managers. IU has been doing most of that" until recently. He mentioned that he had spent the previous few days hosting a huge group of executives from a transnational pharmaceutical company with operations in 120 countries who were considering a major project with AMPATH.

The visit had been set up by Ms. Megan Miller, AMPATH's associate director, and Ms. Teresa Rhodes, the director of development and communications at the IU Center for Global Health in Indianapolis. They had devoted years of effort to managing the relationship between this major supporter and AMPATH. Over that time, they had been able to explain the unique partnership to international organizations in a way that made sense to them. The executives were not used to working directly with Africans, and the IU role was critically important.

Adrian explained that in a future based on the population health model, "you've got to have someone who is a custodian of those relationships on the Kenyan side. Kenyans will need someone with the kind of background Megan has who can manage a donor and explain all of the unique aspects of AMPATH. It's not that Kenyans have not been involved all along, but it requires someone special to talk to foreigners in a way that they understand." He mentioned Beryl Maritim as someone able to explain the relationship just as ably. The young Kenyan had been doing public relations for AMPATH, but by the time I arrived in Eldoret, she was working closely with the Population Health team.

Adrian and I talked quite a bit about the cultural appreciation gained by spending time living abroad—about how living in Eldoret and working so intimately with Kenyans helps him explain to visitors what he knows to be true but that the guests cannot quite yet imagine. "A couple of the people at dinner yesterday said, 'It is just

Facing, The dining hall of IU House, which along with the kitchen takes up the ground floor of house two of the four-house compound, is a favorite place for Bob Einterz. He has shared hundreds of meals here with Hoosiers and other members of the AMPATH Consortium since he first visited Eldoret in 1988. Until 2020, Bob was executive director of the AMPATH Consortium and director of the Indiana University Center for Global Health in Indianapolis. Although his name is near the top of nearly every major grant awarded to the IU-Kenya Partnership, he seemed proudest of having the basketball hoop installed in the courtyard. He is a real Hoosier.

amazing what you and Jess are doing here,' and I thought, 'Well, that's not really the point.' But that's what they can relate to as opposed to, 'It is really great what these Kenyans are doing to bring up their system.' Seeing that requires a depth of understanding that you don't get on the first trip," Adrian explained.

"I see this only with the leadership of companies or donors that have not spent much time here. For some of these people, it's their first trip to Africa. They are struggling to understand what they are seeing. The people that come regularly and know us, they understand why we're putting Kenyans in the lead," he said. "I do not mean to judge them. They are good people. It's just a matter of what they've experienced and what they've seen."

So many Americans' and Europeans' understandings of Africa rest upon an indefensible history that posits that *wazungu* brought enlightenment to the "dark continent." It is still somewhat exceptional to think of foreigners collaborating with Africans as equals in a partnership, rather than acting like saviors from abroad. The "foreign savior" notion has never been the AMPATH approach. The first lesson for all who visit the IU House, the MTRH, and Moi University is that you go to learn in the company of colleagues. I never met a single North American in AMPATH who did not credit Kenyans with being in control of their destiny, and no Kenyan in AMPATH ever told me they thought *wazungu* were here to save them. The "Hoosiers" in Eldoret—whether they are actually from Duke, Toronto, Purdue, Johns Hopkins, or any other consortium university—have always understood AMPATH as a partnership of highly skilled, highly motivated people pursuing good, regardless of where they were born. Over the years, responsibilities have shifted as capacity has been built and Kenyan organizations have matured. But the grounding of the relationships has always been mutual respect and friendship. I see no reason this will

ever change, although AMPATH will clearly continue to evolve.

Adrian was obviously thinking a lot about the future on the afternoon of our interview. It was too early for him to tell me on the record, but he was about to become director of the IU Center for Global Health. By the next February, Bob Einterz had retired, and Adrian moved into Bob's former office in Indianapolis during the spring of IU's bicentennial year in 2020.

As we finished up that day in the Consortium Space, Adrian was reflective. He said,

> One of the things they asked me yesterday was what am I most proud of that AMPATH has achieved. My answer is not what *I* have achieved over the last seven years but what *we* have achieved over the last thirty. It is the "creative resilience." I think that is one of the things that really defines AMPATH differently from other efforts. A lot of these global health partnerships—particularly if they're focused on a specific project run by a couple of individuals working together for a couple of years—they either succeed and those individuals grow bigger than their institution or bigger than their dean or they fail and the whole thing falls apart because money was squandered or something didn't work well and the North American instructions say, "This is too risky, too much risk here." What we've done here at AMPATH is to create a program that can fail, recover, learn from it, and do it again. That is what sustainability is, frankly. And that is what friendship is.

Friendships at AMPATH: never daunted, they cannot falter. This phrase from the IU Hoosier fight song applies to the university's partnership in Kenya as firmly as it applies to IU's commitment to basketball.

Bob Einterz

Most Westerners probably come to know of AMPATH by way of Joe Mamlin, the wise sage who has spent more

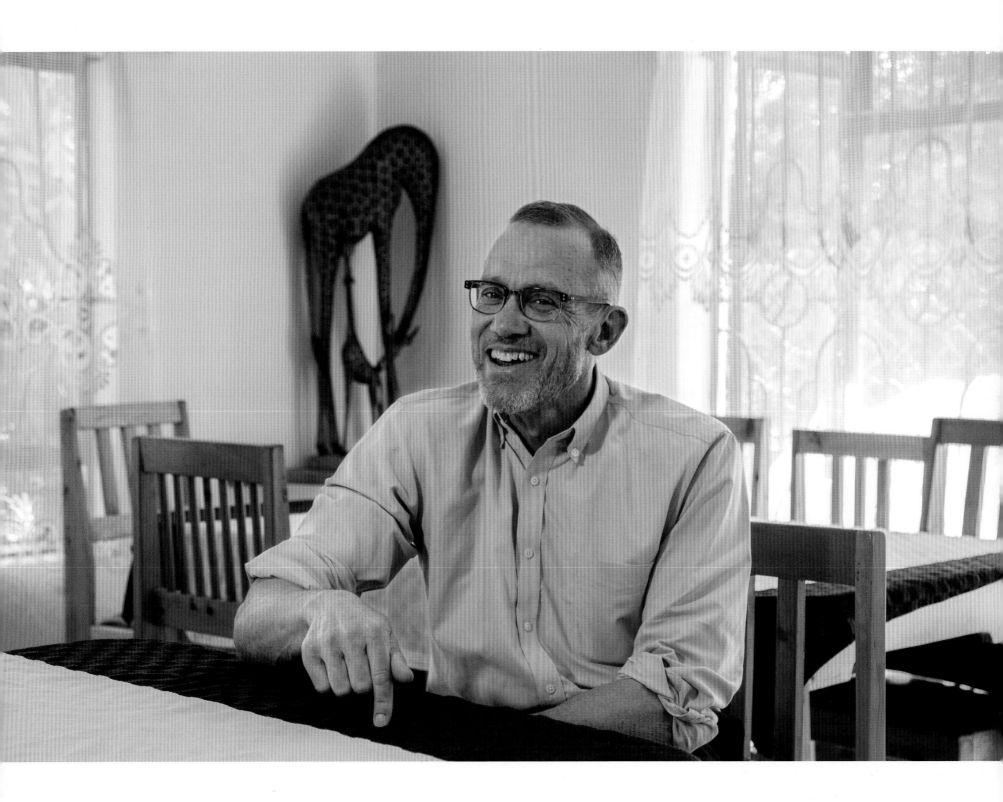

time on the ground in Eldoret than any other North American. Dr. Bob Einterz has always been the other half of the equation at IU. He and Joe were there at the start, visiting Haroun Mengech in 1998 and joining him to create the original partnership between IU and Moi University. Bob's name is near the top of nearly every major grant AMPATH has landed over the years, and his behind-the-scenes negotiations with private and public donors have delivered critically important funding to projects large and small when money was most urgently needed.

When I talked with Bob in December of 2019, he was an associate dean in the IU School of Medicine and director of the IU Center for Global Health, located in a historic building at the center of the Indianapolis medical campus. Upon greeting me at the front door, he explained that we were standing in what once was the Rotary Convalescent Home. It had been built at the height of the polio epidemic to care for children recovering after treatment at the Riley Hospital for Children just across the street. He was obviously proud to work in a building associated with the end of an epidemic.

But Bob is not one to look back very often. He began our conversation by expressing his excitement over new efforts to replicate the AMPATH model:

> To truly replicate the paradigm, we needed to have another North American Academic Health Sciences Center anchor in Ghana and another anchor in Mexico. Our protégés, Dr. Raj Vedanthan, who is at New York University's medical school [NYU], and Dr. Tim Mercer, who is at University of Texas's medical school in Austin [UT], have each formerly served as team leaders in Eldoret. Now they are going to lead those two initiatives with NYU in Ghana and UT in Mexico. The idea is that IU will serve as the overall secretariat of AMPATH Kenya, and soon, if you will, AMPATH Ghana and AMPATH Mexico. And in my mind, because I've never thought that global health

meant that we had to be outside of our own borders, we will not just have three sites, we really have six different sites: Kenya and Ghana and Mexico, and we will have Indiana and New York City and Austin.

Bob did not mention that he and Joe had visited Ghana during their search for a collaborator back in 1988 or that his idea for engaging the US sites is linked to his role as director of the Westside Community Health Center in Indianapolis for nearly ten years. Those were old dreams coming true now because he had been nurturing them for decades. Bob looks forward more than backward, but I had come to Indianapolis to ask him about the early days of the IU-Kenya Partnership and was also thinking of my earliest connection to the project.

In September 2007, my journalism dean had asked me to meet with folks at the medical school in Indianapolis to explore a collaboration in Kenya between the two schools. I arranged a meeting with Fran Quigley in the old Wishard Memorial Hospital building, where AMPATH was then located. Associate dean Bonnie Brownlee joined me for the hour-long drive north. We had a very pleasant meeting with Fran and learned that he was writing a book about the role of Bob and Joe and everyone at IU and Moi in addressing the HIV/AIDS epidemic. That book, *Walking Together, Walking Far* (Quigley 2009), tells how the still-young collaboration between IU and Moi responded to the HIV/AIDS epidemic by growing their partnership into a broad consortium of universities, creating a model program for saving lives, and economically empowering the sick and impoverished. The book is still required reading for the North American medical students and others who travel to Eldoret, and it can be found on most bookshelves in Moi's medical school faculty offices.

But at the time of that first brief meeting, I did not know any of that. I had been running training workshops for East African journalists reporting on HIV/AIDs for five years by then, but I had never heard of AMPATH. As Fran, Bonnie, and I were wrapping up our meeting, Bob stepped into the room to say hello and let us know he was happy we were interested in the partnership with Moi. He was wearing a blue shirt without a coat or tie. I thought he was office staff. I now know he would have been nonplussed by the mischaracterization. Like his partner, Joe, he is so self-effacing and unpretentious that everyone seems his equal, even though his many accomplishments place him in a rarified place few arrive at during their careers.

That brief meeting was a dozen years ago. A lot had changed, and more change was just weeks away as I sat in Bob's corner office. I had waited to interview him until this moment because, while in Eldoret, I had learned that he would be retiring soon. In October 2019, IU president Michael McRobbie awarded Bob the President's Medal for Excellence during a fancy dinner in Indianapolis. It is the highest honor an IU president can bestow. Bob was in that rarified company he had earned.

A month earlier, Bob had officially announced his retirement. He had completed thirty years of teaching at IU at the end of January 2020, and that would be enough. His decision followed the departure of Joe Mamlin from Eldoret in May 2019. Within a year, the two doctors who thirty years earlier had joined with colleagues at Moi University to build a medical school, create a program to treat the HIV/AIDS epidemic, and initiate a population health approach in western Kenya had stepped aside so their protégés could take over.

"This a terrific transition opportunity. We have Adrian Gardner, who has served as the executive field director for seven years. He is wonderfully trained and clearly has much greater equanimity than I have. You know, I like to say that Wabash College is top notch and that we have to dip down a little bit with Adrian's Harvard and Brown degrees, but we'll take it," he said with a mischievous smile and obvious pleasure that the man he had mentored for so long would soon occupy his office. "We have terrific leadership coming in to replace me. Adrian understands the system because he grew up in our system, and he has similarly experienced partners at Moi who are ready to take all this to the next level."

He continued, "I will stay engaged in the secretariat of AMPATH, and if they feel that any of my experience, guidance, and insights can be of help, great! Happy to do that." Bob was still looking to the future, even at the end of his time at the top of the grand project he had started half a lifetime earlier. But I still wanted to learn about the earliest days. I wanted to know how it all started.

When he and I had last met in May, Bob had been in Eldoret hosting some big donors who wanted to meet with the AMPATH leadership. I was able to chat with him in the IU House and then walk with him over to Testimony School, where he was going to take a swim in their pool. Turns out he had been using the school's pool for nearly fifteen years. While it was just a pleasant ten-minute walk for me, it was a bit like going back in time for Bob. As we crossed the bridge over the Sosiani River and walked up the hill, he said, "You know, the original IU House is just around the corner there." He said he would take me there.

The neighborhood is now fully developed, with houses on every lot, but in 1990, when Bob was the first team leader from IU in Eldoret, the home he rented from Mr. Ibrahim Hussein was nearly alone on the slope that led down to the river from Testimony School. Bob and the guests who stayed with him had a twenty-minute walk over to the MTRH and the Moi medical school classrooms. Ibrahim rented the house to IU because he was often out of the country. Two years before, in 1988, Ibrahim had been the first Kenyan to win the Boston Marathon. He had set a world record and was one of the country's leading long-distance runners. It was Ibrahim who began the Kenyan dominance over marathon races that persists to this day. Coincidentally, Eliud Kipchoge, another Kenyan runner from near Eldoret, had broken the elusive "two-hour marathon" record just a few days before Bob announced his retirement (Agence France-Presse 2019). Running is to Kenya as basketball is to Indiana. It's in the blood.

Bob's wife, Ms. Lea Anne Einterz, had lived with Bob in the developing world before Kenya. Five years earlier, during Bob's first year on the IU medical school faculty, they had moved with their two sons to Croix Fer, Haiti, a dusty, desperately poor town just a few kilometers west of the border with the Dominican Republic. Bob had wanted to work in global health, and the Minnesota International Health Volunteers provided him the opportunity. During most of their year in Croix Fer, the Einterz family had no car, no electricity, and no running water.

According to an account in Fran Quigley's book, Bob said, "I learned firsthand about the concept of primary healthcare, a physician's role in the community, and the role of economics and culture in healthcare. We worked on income generation, family planning, and creating mothers' groups. I learned about the critically important role of women in development. Overall, the experience working side-by-side in the community taught me both about the complexity of delivering quality public health and about the importance of community to tackle these problems" (2009, 23).

Those were the lessons he was bringing to Eldoret—the same lessons his friend Joe Mamlin had learned in Afghanistan in the 1960s. By the time the Einterzes had moved into Ibrahim's house, Mengech had a dozen faculty members on staff and the first Moi University medical school class of forty students were ready to begin their studies. Six IU medical students and residents spent time in Kenya that first year, and all spent some time in the big house with Bob and Lea Anne.

Bob spent time running to stay fit. He was a reasonably competitive triathlete for his age group in Indiana but recalled that his running partner, Michael, a student at Testimony School, "made me look like a snail." Together they ran the roads around Eldoret and did wind sprints up the hill to the school. Folks in town no doubt appreciated a *mzungu daktari* (foreign doctor) who could run.

Like most middle-class homes in Kenya, the main house and gardens were surrounded by eight-foot-high walls, not unlike similar neighborhoods in London or other English cities. Remnants of colonialism persist in much of Kenya. The gate leading into the compound was closed and solid, so as we approached, I could only see the rooftop and a tall pine tree on the left just inside. Bob said there were once trees on both sides of the gate but that one afternoon in December of that first year, he had returned home from the hospital to find the tree on the right missing. Lea Anne had taken it inside the house and decorated it for Christmas. "I was sad at the loss of the tree, but it reminded me how far we were from home and how important symbols like an evergreen tree in the house were to a family making a home so far from home," he said. "That's still one of our favorite stories. Eldoret has been home now for thirty years."

I wondered how many more stories there were behind that gate. Eldoret, even in the 1990s, offered far more creature comforts than Haiti. Most of the major streets were paved, the electricity was on most of the time, and there were cars enough to get the school's faculty out to rural clinics like the one in Mosoriot, where they were putting ideas about community-based education and service into practice. It wasn't Indianapolis by any stretch, but it was home.

"The first ten years was a process of building relationships among individuals and institutions," Bob said. "Initially, we were nested within the division general internal medicine. It was just general internists. But soon there were pediatricians and other disciplines within medicine and then subspecialties and sub-subspecialties. We expanded our network beyond the medical school before long because individual relationships have a way of growing when you have strong institutional relationships. Our colleagues in the MTRH joined with us in the med school. That was the genesis, of course, of the AMPATH Consortium, too, which back then we called the Asante consortium"—when other North American universities joined the increasingly strong relationships between physician educators and physician practitioners.

"Because IU relied on funding through philanthropy, we were building relationships within our own community right here in Indiana also," he explained. The faith community in Indianapolis provided assistance, as did many of the foundations in the city and other philanthropic organizations. Just as Kenyans were building institutional relationships between the MTRH, the Ministry of Health, Moi University, and the Ministry of Education, so too were Hoosier institutions coming together in common purpose because of the many personal relationships their members were cultivating.

It wasn't that there was no HIV in Kenya during that first decade, but the epidemic was relatively small and not the nearly overwhelming catastrophe it would become by the start of the second decade. "In fact, one of our very first research projects was headed by Kara Wools and Diana Menya to do research and bring up a lab in the early 1990s focusing on sexually transmitted diseases inclusive

of HIV," he said. The Moi instructional program was famously designed around a problem-based curriculum. "The very first problem given to that first batch of students happened to be about a truck driver traveling from Mombasa to Uganda who presented with swollen lymph nodes," he said. "It was a case of HIV."

Bob and I walked back to the main road and over to Testimony School. The guard at the gate did not recognize Bob, but after a quick phone call to the office, we were let in, and we walked over to the pool past giant candelabra cactuses reaching ten meters into the air. Bob had done this walk dozens, maybe hundreds of times over the years. A lot had changed since his children were toddlers in the old IU House, but some things had stayed the same. I said goodbye and left him to his swim, alone in the outdoor pool just up the street from the pink house where he and his young family had lived when it was all very new.

In May in Kenya, when Bob was telling me these stories about the early days in Eldoret, the weather was warm, the breeze was gentle, and we were in shirtsleeves. But in his Indianapolis office in December, it was just below freezing, snow was in the air, and the idea of swimming outside was unimaginable. Bob sat behind his desk deflecting my questions about the early days and instead continued to talk about the future of AMPATH when suddenly he said, "Just as an aside, there's Joe walking across to Eskenazi Hospital. It is great to see him. He's getting ready to go to Kenya now that his vacation is over." These two Hoosiers somehow think living in Indiana is vacation and living in Eldoret is home.

For North Americans, however, living as residents in Kenya is becoming increasingly formidable and expensive. Since the postelection violence in 2008 that shocked Kenyans into full realization that the tension between tribes had to be eased, politicians and other leaders have made genuine efforts to eliminate the corruption that plagues so many developing countries. In 2011, Kenya enacted a new constitution that devolved power away from the national government in Nairobi to the forty-seven county governments. The Kenya Revenue Authority has become more efficient at collecting taxes. Recent investments in ports and infrastructure financed primarily by Chinese banks, as well as the push toward universal healthcare, have caused the government to redouble its efforts to increase revenues and tighten up regulations on foreigners doing business in the country. As a result, it is becoming harder for members of the AMPATH Consortium to obtain residence visas, and when they do, they are finding that the government wants to tax their salaries as if they were Kenyans. In earlier times, AMPATH could import donated medical equipment into the country duty-free, but tax enforcement now makes that prohibitively expensive.

"It is a delicate matter," Bob explained. Kenyans are developing their country, and taxes are a key mechanism for empowering the government, particularly local county governments, to fund projects focused on needs identified by local people. According to the World Bank, less than 15 percent of Kenya's public expenditures are foreign financed, compared to more than 40 percent in neighboring Uganda and Tanzania. Kenya boasts one of the strongest revenue performances in Africa, and most of Kenya's public services are financed with money from Kenyan taxpayers. The still-recent shift of revenue control from the central government to the counties has further increased the efficiency of the country's development efforts. As a result, the MTRH, Moi University, and AMAPTH are ever more engaged with the county governments in their area. The counties have more fiscal authority over healthcare as expenditures on infrastructure and personnel are increasing.

"As we had expected and as we had hoped, the Kenyan leadership are feeling their oats. And they should. We are very pleased about that. It was never our intention to lead over there, and I would suggest that we never really did lead over there. Our plan was always to work underneath their leadership, Kenyan leadership, and to report to their leadership," Bob stated.

"That said, we did play a significant and instrumental role in the development of the medical school and the health system. But over time, as Kenyans have grown into leadership positions and as the work force has grown, the number of disciplines has expanded, and more and more Kenyans have the education and the experience to run complex operations," he said. The need for *wazungu* on the wards is declining.

"My own thought was that as the relationship evolved, we would become less engaged over decades in the actual delivery of services. And as Kenyans themselves develop not just the expertise but also the wealth that we in the United States have, I imagined it would become a much more equal partnership. And it has. We are now evolving more toward shared training experiences and shared research experiences," Bob concluded.

The partnership has indeed become more equal over the years. Kenyans do have more resources now. They have educated hundreds of doctors at the medical school, and other Kenyan universities and colleges have educated thousands of nurses, technicians, social workers, counselors, and others who work each day to care for the nation's health. But Kenyans still appreciate the help offered by the North Americans, and folks from both sides of the ocean cherish the friendships that have grown over the years.

To me as an outsider, it has been fairly easy to understand why the Kenyans would join in partnership. The wealthier *wazungu* had resources they needed. I do not claim to fully understand their motivations, but folks I talked with told me again and again that they want to build their community and develop their country. That makes sense to me. Their families benefit directly from their efforts.

But what motivates a highly valuable physician to leave a comfortable faculty office in America to devote so much of his or her career to developing someone else's country? I asked Bob.

> I think my motivation to some degree has changed over time. It still comes from my Judeo-Christian heritage, my philosophy, theology, beliefs, and all the usual stuff. We each have certain gifts, certain talents, and we have an obligation to develop those to the best of our ability. And I believe we have an obligation to use those talents to change our world and ourselves for the better. We recognize that we as individuals are flawed and imperfect. We find meaning in life by striving for perfection, all the while recognizing that we will never achieve it. . . . It is the myth of Sisyphus: over and over and over again. Yeah. Putting our shoulder to the boulder and pushing it up the hill. It gives us meaning and satisfaction. It is what we should be doing.
>
> My belief system and philosophy haven't changed a whole lot over the years, but I think I am far more cognizant and aware of my own flaws and my own imperfections than I was thirty-five years ago. I want to say that I am far more tolerant in some ways now. I think I am more discerning of the complexity of individuals and communities and relationships. I see far more shades of gray. In fact, it is probably rare to say that I see in black and white anymore. Almost everything tends to be shades of gray.

"But," he concluded, "I do still believe that there is this absolute good. It is love. And so, there is the motivation. It is love.

At the end of January 2020, just a few days after IU celebrated its two-hundred-year anniversary, Bob retired from the university he had shaped so profoundly. He and his wife moved their home again—this time to South Bend, Indiana, where Lea Anne has family. It was only the two of them this time, no toddlers. They settled into a house they own that has central heating, reliable electricity, and two cars in the garage. As always, Bob goes to work every day to put the lessons he has learned in global heath into practice, but now it is as the chief health officer for Saint Joseph County.

Honestly, he went to work for Saint Joseph County. "Saint Joe" and Bob—together even in retirement.

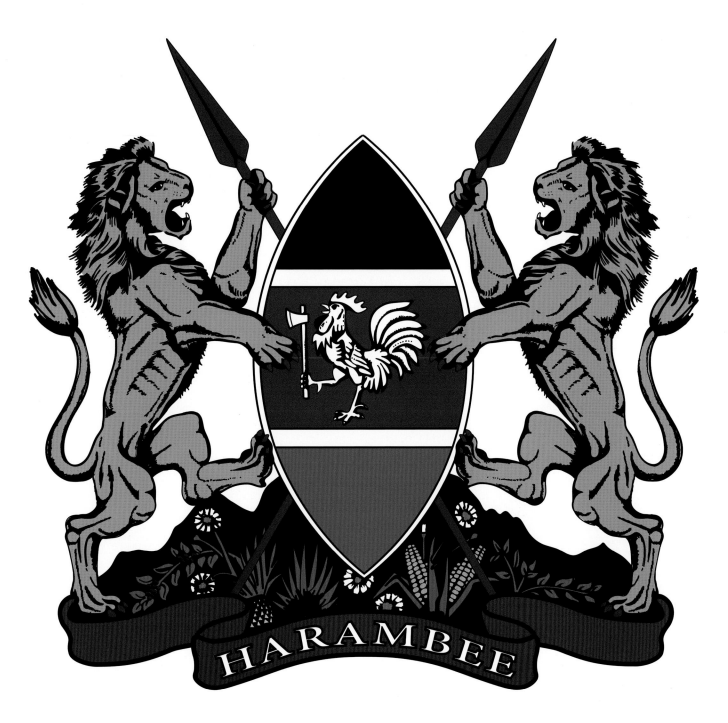

The Kenyan Coat of Arms features the Swahili word *harambee*, which translates to English as, "let's all pull together."

PART FOUR

RESEARCH

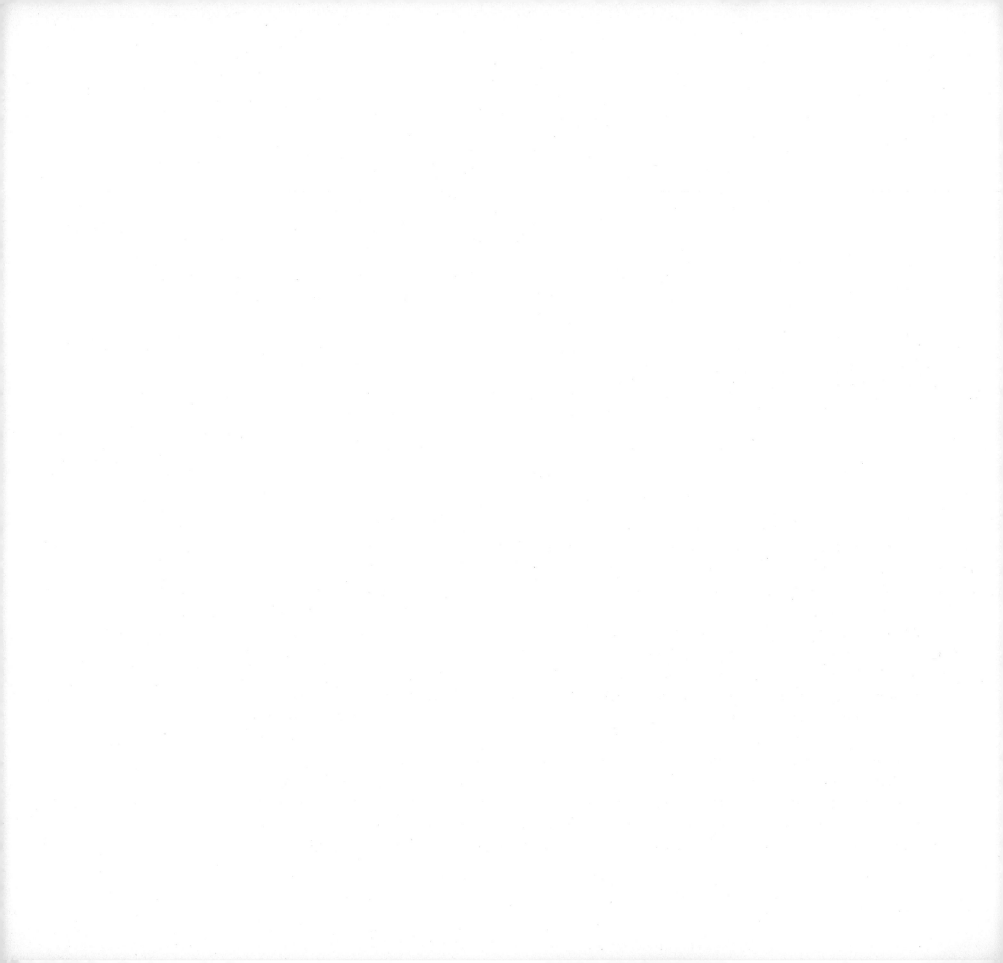

CHAPTER NINE

Methodology

My education and professional experience are in journalism. I started working for my small town's newspaper when I was sixteen. I studied journalism as an undergraduate at West Virginia University, began my working career as a photojournalist for the Associated Press, and finished my professional career at the *South Bend Tribune* in Indiana. I then studied journalism in graduate school at Indiana University and graduated from Bloomington with a doctorate that had prepared me for research in social science. I have a deep appreciation for the insight that photojournalism can reveal though the intimate observation of people, and I have a deep respect for the insight that scientifically prescribed methods can discern. In this book, I combined the two to create a document that touches the reader's emotion and intellect—heart and mind. I hope this method is persuasive to both an academic audience interested in advancing general knowledge about the role of worker motivation in healthcare performance outcomes and a lay audience interested in knowing about how health workers feel about who they are and why they work so hard to build their society.

My approach to the photography has been fundamentally journalistic. I selected my participants because they struck me as people with a good story to tell and an ability to express themselves freely and clearly. Except for the portraits, none of the photos were posed or directed. Like a photojournalist, I spent dozens of hours and thousands of exposures trying to capture candid moments of unscripted behavior. I spent enough time with every subject that they came to almost forget I was there and paid little attention to the fact that I was making photos. The result was a series of stories told primarily with photos. I wrote down quotations and observations for the captions, but the narrative thread that connects the beginning, middle, and end of each of the eight stories is visual rather than textual. This photo story approach has its origins in the great photo magazines of the 1930s like *LIFE* and *LOOK* but is well practiced at newspapers and magazines around the world now. I modified that basic approach because I had the luxury of time and am therefore more confident that I have told stories that ring true to the subject as well as the reader.

I supplemented my photojournalism approach with visual sociology techniques often used by anthropologists called photo elicitation. Because anthropologists are uncertain about how their own cultural backgrounds influence their understanding of other cultural practices, they make photographs of those practices and use them to elicit comments from the folks they are trying to understand. In sociology and anthropology, the findings are what the participants say in response to the photographs. The photos may or may not be of the participants or even of their surroundings. The photos function as tools that encourage explanation by participants. Visuals are used to understand things that are not easily put in words, especially when the researcher and the subject speak different languages. The visual becomes something of a translation device.

However, I was interested in whether the healthcare workers I was observing agreed with me that the images I was capturing were true representations of their efforts. It was their story that I was trying to tell, after all. I am not African or Kenyan. *Wazungu* stand out in even the largest crowds in Eldoret. A *mzungu* who is 6'3", sixty-two years old, and carrying a camera worth a year's salary for many

AMPATH workers stood out even more. Far too many of the people I photographed in the past had felt abused by foreigners with cameras. They had been photographed by tourists in moving cars or had found foreigners taking photos of their children without permission. I did not want to be that *mzungu* who took photos Kenyans would look at with disappointment because the photographer was culturally insensitive and had made them out to be something they are not. If I was going to tell their story, it had to be a story they recognized as their own.

I consulted with the public relations team at AMPATH and MTRH and eventually identified four stories to pursue. AMPATH has about fifty projects ongoing most of the time these days—more than anyone could confidently list. I identified four that had a long history but were undergoing innovations that point to the future of AMPATH. The first was about Anyara Papa, a microfinance specialist who had been with AMPATH since the very start and was working on an economic-empowerment project aimed at persuading villagers to enroll in the National Hospital Insurance Fund as a way of sustainably ensuring that they could pay for necessary healthcare. The second was about Pamela Were, an oncology nurse who joined the hospital in Eldoret before it became MTRH and was organizing free cancer-screening clinics in villages across Kenya when I met her. She was applying lessons learned from caring for patients with HIV to another set of previously neglected diseases.

The third story was about two people: one an AMPATH agricultural extension officer and the other a visiting fellow with an international agro-science company. Together, they were working to enhance dairy farmers' production levels by introducing them to scientific feeding practices. This sort of private-public partnership is how AMPATH will increasingly engage external funding for the area's development efforts. The fourth story was not so much about an individual or even a pair of people; it was about a place. Since the early days of comprehensive care for HIV patients, AMPATH has run clinics where clients can receive care that includes antiretroviral therapy, mental health counseling, economic-empowerment referral, and more. The Rafiki Centre is a special clinic open only to adolescents. Located separately from the other comprehensive care clinics on the MTRH campus, Rafiki provides care specifically suited to the special needs of patients who have been HIV positive their entire lives, as well as to those who may be HIV negative but have grown up in a world heavily influenced by the epidemic. There were other stories I might have told, but these seemed to address the ways AMPATH is most significantly moving: sustainable healthcare financing, chronic disease management, economic self-sufficiency, and comprehensive care without stigma.

After every photo session, I reviewed my images and selected a few dozen that were representative. The next time I was with the workers, I showed them the photos on a tablet I carried with me and asked if my photos were true. Was I telling their story? Was I telling it completely? Were the images culturally sensitive? Did I have it right? This was hardly a traditional photojournalistic approach. Journalists do not allow their sources to critique their reporting before publication. But I believe my method empowered the participants in a way that decreased their tendency to do things they thought I wanted and instead gave them license to be themselves in front of the foreigner's camera. It allowed the workers and me to be more honest and deliberate without being artificial and posed. Much of that honesty derives from the fact that we were making these photo stories as collaborating partners. That is the AMPATH way, after all.

My social science research method was also informed by previous social science research. One way to learn from

somebody is to observe them. Photographs allow me to share my observations with others. Another way to learn from somebody is to ask them questions and write down their answers. This too sounds like journalism—and it is. But just as my photojournalism approach was enhanced by modification using an academic research method, so too my questions were similarly informed by a social science method. And on this, I can point directly to a study done a dozen years ago by AMPATH researchers.

In 2006, Professor Tom Inui and his colleagues (2007) wanted to know how AMPATH had managed to use the resources provided by PEPFAR and other donors to so effectively meet the challenge of the HIV epidemic in western Kenya. They used a method called "Appreciative Inquiry" and conducted semi-structured, in-depth interviews of twenty-six AMPATH workers. The key question was, What are some of the most important reasons you continue to work for AMPATH? They concluded that the workers themselves were "the critical assets of an effective program" (1,745). These people's work values and motivations had made a success of a complex academic model, and they had made it work spectacularly well in a most challenging setting. The professors had thought up a model, and the workers had given it life. The professors came to realize this by carefully recording the interviews, generating field notes by independent reviewers, and subjecting those notes to close-reading qualitative analysis for themes. Their research rang clear to me. Their conclusions matched my own observations and corresponded with the reporting my students had done a few years afterward. They had tapped into the motivations that animated the mainline workers at AMPATH.

AMPATH's success has much to do with the contributions of hundreds of similarly dedicated workers who work directly with clients to build personal relationships that provide care that exceeds what medication alone can provide. But their success is in no small part the result of exceptional leadership from those at the top of the organizational charts at the MTRH, the Moi University School of Medicine, and the AMPATH Consortium. Seeing how workers do their work helps us understand the daily mission. Talking to the leadership gives us a sense of why the collaboration among these three organizations works so effectively. Rather than interviewing additional workers, I instead interviewed several of the top leaders in the AMPATH collaboration.

Again, I talked with the public relations folks and identified eleven leaders to interview. Some were obvious because they had been there at the start of the IU-Kenya Partnership and remained influential thirty years later. Others were equally obvious because they headed one of the three organizations in the collaboration. The rest seemed poised to take on greater responsibility as those senior leaders retire. I surely missed someone, but such is the nature of a purposive sample. For every interview, I first asked where they would feel most comfortable talking with me. It was usually an office, but in one case it was an automobile and in others it was in a home. I asked everyone the same three questions. The first was taken from the Inui study: How did you first come to be involved with AMPATH? The other two were modified but tap into the same sentiments: Why has AMPATH succeeded? What motivates you and your team?

And then I asked all these folks if I had gotten it right, just as I had with those in my photo stories. Each person confirmed their quotations and let me know whether the story rang true to them. I used their feedback to modify what I heard in their answers. The essays that appear beside their portraits in chapter 8 are informed both by what they said and what they meant to say.

Finally, as a check on the generalizability of my observations of these individuals to the entire AMPATH workforce, I distributed a survey to the approximately 1,500 members of AMPATH's staff via email. Participants anonymously responded to an online form. The questionnaire contained twenty-one closed-ended questions used to generate three scales measuring the meaning of work, job satisfaction, and commitment to the organization, as well as seven open-ended questions collecting demographics and opinion. Using conventional survey research methods, I reported the frequencies and descriptive statistics and then made some simple cross tabulations that allowed me to speculate in the discussion and conclusion chapter about whether and how the folks I photographed and interviewed accurately represented the workforce of AMPATH.

Was all this necessary? Obviously I think it was, because I do not think readers can really understand the conditions in which these workers perform their duties without at least seeing it with their own eyes. I wish I could let you smell and feel Africa too, but seeing these photos is far more intimate and emotionally captivating than simply reading the words I might have used to describe them. But photo stories, no matter how compelling, are not enough on their own to provide you with a complete story. Africa is filled with storytellers, and a book about them without their words is incomplete. And finally, a good survey provides an empirical observation that liberates a population from its ability or inability to tell a story by giving everyone an opportunity to have a say, at least on a few important questions. Journalism is good at telling stories about what people do, and social science is good at generating theory about how things work. By putting these two approaches together, I hope I have allowed AMPATH workers to tell a story about how they work.

CHAPTER TEN

Staff Responses to the Survey

From the very start of my quest for approval to conduct academic research in Kenya, I was an odd duck. All universities in the US have institutional review boards that oversee research conducted on human subjects. The reason they do so has everything to do with abuse of subjects—particularly African American subjects—by unethical researchers in the past.

James H. Jones (1993) described the experiment most often referenced to explain why academic research must be carefully monitored and approved by peer review:

> From 1932 to 1972, the United States Public Health Service conducted a non-therapeutic experiment involving over 400 black male sharecroppers infected with syphilis. The Tuskegee Study had nothing to do with treatment. Its purpose was to trace the spontaneous evolution of the disease in order to learn how syphilis affected black subjects.

The men were not told they had syphilis; they were not warned about what the disease might do to them; and, with the exception of a smattering of medication during the first few months, they were not given health care. Instead of the powerful drugs they required, they were given aspirin for their aches and pains. Health officials systematically deceived the men into believing they were patients in a government study of "bad blood," a catch-all phrase black sharecroppers used to describe a host of illnesses. At the end of this 40-year deathwatch, more than 100 men had died from syphilis or related complications.

On July 25, 1972, Associated Press reporter Jean Heller published a news story about the experiment that rocked the US medical establishment. Her reporting caused a public outcry that led the assistant secretary for health and scientific affairs to appoint an ad hoc advisory panel

173

to identify the basic ethical principles that should underlie the conduct of biomedical and behavioral research involving human subjects and develop guidelines to assure that such research is conducted in accordance with those principles. Shamefully, such unethical experimentation was much more frequently done on African Americans in the US, part and parcel of racist attitudes in the medical community and in society generally, according to medical ethicist Harriet Washington (2006).

The result of these abuses was the National Research Act of 1974, which mandated that research associated with US universities must be reviewed and found in compliance with ethical practices that demonstrate respect for persons, beneficence, justice, informed consent, and transparent assessment of risks. Indiana University had a long-established protocol for ensuring that research was done ethically, and Moi University established an equally rigorous system to ensure that participants were safe when the medical school was being formed. Meslin, Ayuku, and Were (2014) reported that since 1993, the Moi College of Health Sciences and the MTRH have administered the Institutional Research and Ethics Committee (IREC). It monitors the approval process and reviews hundreds of proposals each year from physician researchers working out of the MTRH.

My research was not medical. I was not administering drugs, drawing blood, or testing new treatments on hospital patients. I just wanted to ask the AMPATH employees whether they liked their job. I wanted to see if the devotion to duty and the job satisfaction I had seen while photographing and interviewing folks like Pamela Were, Kenneth Malaba, and Anyara Papa was generally true of all 1,500 employees or whether I was being told what I wanted to hear. The Institutional Review Board (IRB) in Bloomington routinely deals with requests from social scientists who want to do survey research. Because

participation in my proposed survey was voluntary, and because respondents' identities would not be revealed, my proposal was reviewed and approved in less than a week.

The IREC in Eldoret took a bit longer. And it is good that it did because the history of *wazungu* coming into Africa and acting without ethical regard for the people subjected to their research aims is not always pretty. Media accounts often say that Africans have historically been duped into participation in medical experimentation without appropriate informed consent, and they have, but the history is actually more nuanced. Graboyes said that Africans were "rarely passive recipients of medical interventions . . . but active contributors in the medical encounter" (2015, 8). She stated that because historically there was "no shared sense of what constituted research or why it was done, researchers and participants both tended to talk about these encounters in a transactional way, as a form of exchange" (9). Africans under colonial rule desired modern medical treatment and submitted to research demands to get it—most times to their benefit, but sometimes to their peril. Such is no longer the case. The IREC and the Kenyan MoH have established careful procedures to ensure that research today is done ethically and have trained a bureaucracy to enforce this.

It took nearly three months for my proposal to be approved, but once it was, I was able to move very quickly. Sylvester Kimaiyo told me that Mr. Agustine Miencha in the OpenMRS office would provide me an email list of all AMPATH employees. I walked into Agustine's office just two days before my departure from Eldoret. He greeted me warmly. I told him all about my project: who I had interviewed, who I had photographed, and all the places I had been trying to learn about AMPATH. He seemed pleased by my interest in AMPATH and my professed love of Stoney, the brand of soda pop sitting on his desk.

Stoney is a regional ginger beer that I have loved since my first trip to East Africa. Usually, at the end of a day spent at the MTRH, I would sit on a bench just a few yards from the hospital campus under a roadside umbrella cart run by a kind woman named Salina and drink a Stoney.

Agustine needed a little time to collect everything, so I said I would return the next day. Upon arriving at his small office on the back side of the AMPATH Centre, I handed him a USB drive and he handed it back to me with what I had waited so long for: 1,561 entries on a spreadsheet. There were no names and no job titles, just 1,561 email addresses. Some were the official work address, @ampath.or.ke, but most were Gmail, Yahoo, and other personal accounts. These were the perfect strangers I would ask to share their opinions about the organization they worked for and the work they did to build community. I would do so from my IU office back in Bloomington, because that Tuesday was my last full day in Eldoret. After saying goodbye to some of the friends I had made on the MTRH campus, I walked to my house in Elgon View for the last time. And I stopped to have a Stoney with Salina under her umbrella by the side of Nandi Road.

The rest of this chapter describes the questions I asked in the survey, the method I used to collect the responses, and the techniques I used to analyze the data it yielded. For those who like to read research, you know what to expect. For those of you already tired of IRBs, IRECs, and academic procedures, please skip ahead to the subhead, "Discussion."

Questionnaire Design and Administration of Survey Instrument

My fundamental questions for the survey were whether AMPATH workers professed a commitment to the organization, found satisfaction in the work, believed the work they did was meaningful, and understood their motivation. The literature informing these questions comes primarily from organizational behavior scholars who have studied the potential benefits of meaningful work, both to the individual and to the organizations they work for, as well as older ideas like satisfaction, commitment, and motivation.

Rosso, Dekas, and Wrzesniewski defined meaningful work "not as simply whatever work means to people (meaning), but as work that is both significant and positive in valence (meaningfulness). Furthermore, we add that the positive valence of MW [meaningful work] has a eudaimonic (growth- and purpose-oriented) rather than a hedonic (pleasure-oriented) focus" (2010, 93).

Steger, Dik, and Duffy argued that "many people want their careers and their work to be more than simply a way to earn a paycheck or pass their time; they want their work to mean something" (2012, 1). They developed a Work and Meaning Inventory (WAMI) composed of ten items where respondents answer using a five-point Likert-type scale ranging from "absolutely untrue" to "absolutely true." The WAMI was positively related to desirable work variables (organizational citizenship behaviors, career commitment, organizational commitment, job satisfaction, and intrinsic work motivations) and negatively related to undesirable work variables (days reported absent, withdrawal intentions, and extrinsic work motivations). Their testing demonstrated concurrent and incremental validity.

Because I was particularly interested in job satisfaction and organizational commitment, I also employed two scales to measure these work variables. Both were positively related to the WAMI. To measure job satisfaction, I used the Michigan Organizational Assessment Questionnaire Job Satisfaction Subscale (MOAQJSS) (Cammann et al. 1979), a three-item scale where respondents answer using a five-point Likert-type scale ranging from "strongly disagree" to "strongly agree." Research on job satisfaction has a long history in industrial and organizational psychology, but there is still no single measure that is widely recognized as applicable to all situations. Because of the known correlation between job satisfaction and the WAMI, I chose this simple subscale to measure the concept separately. A recent meta-analysis by Bowling and Hammond (2008) found it reliable and the construct valid.

Commitment to organization has generally been studied as a way to decrease turnover. My interest was to see whether the devotion to task that I witnessed in the field was true for AMPATH's staff generally or whether I had been steered toward outliers by the public relations folks. Certainly, the people I observed were exceptional, but how different were they from their colleagues? Allen and Meyer's (1990) model measures three component parts of the concept: the affective component refers to employees' emotional attachment to, identification with, and involvement in the organization. The continuance component refers to commitment based on the costs that employees associate with leaving the organization, and the normative component refers to employees' feelings of obligation to remain with the organization.

I used only the items measuring the affective component since my interest was in testing to see whether the expressed affection for AMPATH that I had heard from staff in the field was widespread throughout the organization. Like the MOAQJSS, Allen and Meyer's Affective Commitment scale's eight items asked respondents to reply using a five-point Likert-type scale ranging from "strongly disagree" to "strongly agree."

Cronbach's alpha tests were done to test the internal consistency of each of the three scales. Results indicated that all had good reliability: the WAMI produced an alpha

of .810 (ten items); the Job Satisfaction scale was .719 (three items), and the Affective Commitment scale was .789 (eight items). Given that all three scales are widely used measures of the constructs, no items were removed. For presentation, the scales were recoded into quartiles and labeled "very low, low, high, and very high."

I also wanted to test whether responses differed significantly according to how long staff had worked for AMPATH (tenure), whether they identified as men or women (gender), whether they were young or old (age), and whether they were highly educated or not (education). In other words, were these attitudes toward the organization widespread or resident only in a subset of the workforce?

The final question was open-ended and of my own design: What is the main motivation for your work?

The questionnaire therefore was made up of twenty-eight items: twenty-one closed-ended Likert-type statements (six reverse coded), six open-ended demographic questions, and one open-ended question about motivation.

As a final check, my Fulbright supervisor, Dr. Abraham Mulwo of Moi's Department of Communication Studies, reviewed the questionnaire and found it appropriate and accurate. I next consulted with Dr. Jessica Ruff, the population health informatics team lead at Indiana University while I was in Eldoret, about distribution and decided that a Google Form would be the easiest since most Kenyans use Android mobile phones for online access. Jessica said that her team had had the fewest problems with Google Forms.

I posted the survey on July 24, 2019, and, as a pilot test, sent requests to thirty addresses randomly selected from the population list of 1,562. Email addresses were placed in the blind carbon copy field and sent from and to my

Indiana University address. This way, no addresses were shared with any potential respondents. By August 1, I had received four completed questionnaires and six emails. Four messages were from the respondents' servers saying the message was not delivered. One person said he was no longer with AMPATH, and another thanked me for asking her opinion.

Upon examining the four error messages, I discovered what appeared to be data entry errors. I edited the addresses (removing an extra *Y* from a Yahoo address and removing an extra period from a Gmail address) on the master list. This would be my routine throughout the survey period. On August 6, I sent a reminder to the twenty-five addresses that had not completed the questionnaire. Six more completed the questionnaire, and no error messages were generated. The Google form automatically collected respondent email address. I noticed that two had come from addresses I had not sent to. In both cases, the first portion of the address was the same as on my list, but the server was different, suggesting the person had shifted from using Yahoo to Gmail. In cases like this, I edited my master list so no follow-up messages were sent to the old addresses. Because the pilot test indicated no problem with the distribution technique or questionnaire responses, I included the eight responses in the final data set. On August 24, I sent the request to the entire list.

That message generated 132 error replies from servers. I edited addresses for typos and resent the invitation. I sent reminders to nonrespondents on August 29 and September 9. By the end of the collection period, on September 24, I had 125 undeliverable addresses. Sixteen people had responded to the survey from different addresses. Two told me they had left AMPATH. Four people asked me to remove them from my list, with one saying, "I do not trust you." I responded to all four, saying that I would do as requested. I explained to the woman who expressed distrust that, contrary to her assumption, I had actually spent five months talking with AMPATH staff. I reassured her that no individual would be identified and that no one in AMPATH would be aware of her participation or nonparticipation. She completed the survey the next day.

A total of 360 Google forms were completed. Seven people submitted multiple times, likely due to the fact that I requested their participation using one email address and they replied using another. Therefore, when I asked nonparticipants to complete the survey, these individuals again responded since I had not removed their original addresses from the request. In every case, the first response was kept and subsequent responses were removed from the data set. In the end, there were 346 usable responses. The response rate was 24 percent (1,562 − 125 = 1,437 presumed valid email addresses; 346 ÷ 1,437 = 24.08 percent response rate). Three completed the quantitative portion but not the qualitative. Otherwise, there were very few missing values.

Survey research is a tool used to collect information about a well-defined population of persons, like the AMPATH staff, but the reliability of results is vulnerable to three sources of error: sampling error, sample bias, and nonsampling error. I surveyed all staff (census), so there was little possibility of sampling error or sample bias. Nonsampling error is a threat, however, and many analysts argue that a high response rate is a necessary condition for survey validity (American Association for Public Opinion Research n.d.). Survey response rates have declined steadily over the last twenty years, a trend acknowledged by public and private organizations. For example, Kennedy and Hartig (2019) of the Pew Research Center reported that between 2001 and 2018, typical telephone survey response rates in the US fell from 28 percent to just

6 percent. In their words, "While the Center's telephone survey protocol is somewhat different from those used by other organizations, conversations with contractors and other pollsters confirm that the pattern reported here is being experienced more generally in the industry" (1).

A survey of an organization like AMPATH in Kenya differs from the general population surveys done by Pew in the US, of course. Little research has been published about response rates in Kenya, but a recent meta-analysis of organizational research journals published in the US showed that the average response rate for studies utilizing data collected from organizations was 35.7 percent with a standard deviation of 18.8 (Baruch and Holtom 2008). So, while my 24 percent response rate is not outside the range accepted by academic journals, the reliability of the findings here do pose a threat to validity. In Kenya, accessing a web survey entails costs on the part of the respondent since many AMPATH staffers access the Internet via their mobile phones, paying for data in increments as small as KSh 200 (US$2). This may have discouraged participation of lower-paid staffers. Although my email request specifically promised anonymity, staff who believed they were vulnerable may have declined simply because I was associated with their bosses. It is also possible that email addresses I presumed were valid were not actually being monitored by the respondents. After the survey closed, I received twelve messages that said they did not often check the account I had used and apologized for being late in response.

Some assurance of the survey's reliability comes from a large-scale experimental replication by Scott Keeter and colleagues in 2006 that concluded, "Within the limits of the experimental conditions, nonresponse did not introduce substantial biases into the estimates" (777). Less than perfect response is not desirable, but it likely did not seriously threaten the quality of this survey's estimates of staff attitudes. Quantitative data in this study were processed and analyzed using IBM SPSS Statistics (version 25).

Findings

The average respondent was thirty-five years old (mean = 34.97, std dev = 7.54) and had worked for AMPATH for five years (mean = 4.98, std dev = 5.13). It is likely that many had worked for the MoH for longer than this, but my interest was in staff members' thoughts about AMPATH, not the larger health organization, as interesting as that might be. Almost as many men responded as did women (50.6% female, 49.4% male). Robert Rono, head of AMPATH's RSPO, said that in August 2019, 55.1% of all employees were women, and the average age was 36.4. The survey results are therefore similar to the population, at least on these two measures.

Difference of means tests were conducted on all three scales to determine if responses were statistically different according to gender. A Student's t-test using independent samples assuming equal variance indicated no significant difference (WAMI $t = 1.09$, $df = 338$, two-tailed significance = .276; Job Satisfaction $t = -.112$, $df = 338$, two-tailed significance = .911; Affective Commitment $t = .880$, $df = 336$, two-tailed significance = .379). Pearson correlation coefficients were calculated for the three scales and age, tenure, and education. None were significant at $p \leq .05$. It is reasonable to assume that staff assessment of their workplace did not differ according to gender, age, tenure, or education level.

The range for all three scales was 1 to 4. The mean response to the Work and Meaning Inventory was 3.83 (std dev = .43), the mean response to the Job Satisfaction scale was 3.40 (std dev = .77), and the mean response to the Affective Commitment scale was 3.20 (std dev = .75).

More than 85 percent of respondents were in the top quartile, or "very high," on the WAMI, 54 percent were "very high" on job satisfaction, and 37 percent were "very high" on Affective Commitment.

Discussion

The percentage of respondents scoring high or very high on all three scales is startling. Only 6 people of 346 (1.7%) scored low on the Work and Meaning Inventory, only 37 people (10.7%) were low on Job Satisfaction, and just 45 (13%) were low on their Affective Commitment to AMPATH. Or, to put it positively, 93 percent of the staffers indicated they found a high level of meaning in their work, 89 percent were highly satisfied with their job, and 86 percent were highly committed to AMPATH as an organization. The enthusiasm for their work and the commitment I witnessed as I watched dozens of staff interact with clients over the five months I observed them in informal situations appear to be the norm and not some artifact of my interaction with the public relations staff or the North Americans who live and work in Eldoret.

The purpose of the survey was to test whether the anecdotal evidence I had collected from the leadership and the staff working in area communities was representative of the average AMPATH staffer. These results strongly suggest that my reporting was valid. As I admitted early on, I am not an organizational behavior expert, and I did not collect information on enough variables to suggest *why* AMPATH workers are as satisfied and committed as they are. I suspect the 24 percent response rate would have been lower if I had asked more probing questions about specific financial incentives, career development, and management issues—maybe because they are even more sensitive but maybe because a longer survey simply costs respondents more money. Mobile phone data is not free.

That said, comparison to other studies of East African healthcare workers is instructive. Retention has historically been a serious problem across the region, including Kenya. The demand for skilled nurses in the West has contributed to considerable outmigration from Kenya over the last few decades despite severe need for their services. In 2013, the World Health Organization (WHO) estimated that although sub-Saharan Africa had 25 percent of the world's diseases burden, it possessed only 1.3 percent of the trained health workforce. The ratio of practicing nurses to population in Kenya in 2015 was 8.3 nurses per 10,000 population compared with the WHO recommendation of 25 nurses per 10,000. Kenya had 5,660 doctors and 603 dentists retained in the country, which translated to approximately 1.5 doctors and 0.2 dentists to 10,000 population, against the WHO recommended minimum staffing level of 36 doctors per 10,000 population (MoH 2015b). Another government report noted that "Kenya currently faces significant challenges in overcoming health worker shortages and low retention, as well as difficulty in attaining equitable distribution of human resources for health—particularly in hard-to-reach areas" (MoH 2015a, 5). Eldoret is one of those areas.

A 2008 metastudy by Willis-Shattuck analyzed twenty qualitative and quantitative articles that examined the motivation and retention of health workers in developing countries. The study noted that health worker retention is critical for health system performance and that motivation is key to retention. It concluded that while financial incentives, career development, and management issues are core factors, they are not enough, and adequate resources and appropriate infrastructure can improve morale significantly. Recall that MTRH CEO Aruasa pointed to very high retention figures when I asked him about the challenge of keeping his highly skilled workers in Kenya, and he said the partnership between the Ministry of Health and AMPATH had achieved this by providing the resources and innovative organizational infrastructure staff need to thrive.

Job satisfaction is ultimately dependent upon these factors. A 2014 study examined motivation and retention of 404 healthcare workers in three disparate regions in Kenya and provides some comparison to the findings here since they did measure job satisfaction. Job satisfaction was considerably lower than at AMPATH, with just 46 percent of respondents at high or very high levels compared to 89.3 percent at AMPATH. Interestingly, when asked if they would take a job outside of Kenya if given the opportunity, 72 percent of that study's respondents said they would (Ojakaa, Olango, and Jarvis 2014). This comparison is fraught since the job satisfaction scales were not identical. I didn't ask about the desirability of out-migration, and the regions they surveyed were Turkana, Machakos, and Kibera—not Eldoret. But the relative difference between 46 and 72 percent nevertheless suggests that the high levels of satisfaction observed at AMPATH are not common across the country.

My findings are also not surprising given the results of a 2007 study led by Tom Inui at the Regenstrief Institute in Indianapolis and colleagues at IU and Moi. They asked twenty-six AMPATH staff about why their organization was succeeding so spectacularly. The structured interviews revealed that employees perceived themselves as "creating effectively, connecting with others, making a difference, serving those in great need, providing comprehensive care to restore healthy lives, and growing as a person and a professional" (Inui et al. 2007, 1,745).

These same themes were evident in the responses to a qualitative question I asked: What is the main motivation for your work? Unlike Inui and colleagues, I did not do a systematic analysis, but the answers I present here are not atypical: Dozens mentioned reliable salary and quality training, strong leadership, and past achievements, but the most common comment was something about "seeing the patients get better and serving the community." More specifically, of the 342 people who answered the question, 49 mentioned "salary" or "pay," 56 mentioned "service," and 142 mentioned "client," "patient," or "community." Some of the more illuminating responses are instructive beyond these simple counts.

For example, a nutrition and dietetics officer said, "AMPATH's consistency in payment motivates me a lot and also makes me to trust them because they are faithful employers." As did several others, she tied salary to faith in the organization. A clinical nurse said she was motivated most by "teamwork and support from my AMPATH Plus family." An adherence nurse said she found motivation "when my clients are satisfied with the services I offer, which can bring positive impact on their daily lives." A sustainability assistant said her motivation was "helping the less fortunate, providing for my family, teaching the community the importance of testing/screening, empowering people around me, giving life skills to AMPATH clients," while a clinical officer said it was "giving hope to the clients I interact with every day" and a subordinate staff member said it was "seeing that the organization achieve its goals and successfully runs its operation on healthcare services."

One sustainability assistant said he liked "being a living testimony. I share my story to those who have lost hope after knowing their status. Then, working together, I see those families rise again and I get encouraged." An AMPATH Plus clinician said he was sustained by "seeing adolescents who were born positive grow healthily by accepting their status and taking their ARVs well." An HIV testing services counselor said, "I have bosses who are always there for me, they encourage me a lot," and a medical social worker said she was encouraged by "trainings and performance-based incentives."

Conclusion

These survey findings cannot be used to refine a construct or test a theory. While that is the goal in much of the academic research that I and other academics perform, my goal for the survey was more simply to provide confirmation that what I had seen during the five months I spent living in Eldoret and watching a few dozen AMPATH workers engage with their clients, patients, and communities was representative of the entire operation. I think it has provided solid evidence that the chapters that precede this one are more than just the haphazard observations of a *mzungu* who was directed toward a story by public relations officers and later walked away with an impression based on what he wanted to see. Instead, I interpret these kind responses from nearly a quarter of the people who make AMPATH a success as confirmation that my reporting and photographic methods yielded insights that are typical and representative of the thousands of successful outcomes generated by a healthcare workforce that is devoted to its community and has the supports necessary to perform quality care—day in and day out.

CHAPTER ELEVEN

Discussion and Conclusions

No *mzungu* should write about Africa without the words of Binyavanga Wainaina ringing in their head. The Kenyan author's satiric essay, "How to Write About Africa" (2005), is a long list of the objectifying platitudes that characterize so much of what has been and is still written about Africa by Westerners: those who visit a game park and depart, those who parachute in to report on a war, and those who spend a research sabbatical. For me, it was initially a painful read. I was not immune to stereotypes and tropes, but Wainaina helped me laugh at myself and, I think, look at Africa more empathetically.

As I sit down to write this final chapter, I also have the words of a Cameroonian health policy consultant ringing in my head. Desmond Jumbam's recent editorial in *BMJ*

Global Health (2020) offers a similarly satiric set of admonitions about how to conduct medical research and write up one's results that is also a primer on what not to do. He warns us not to ignore the real experts: the Africans who treat the patients, conduct the research, and know healthcare in Africa by way of both scholarship and life experience. Like Wainaina, his Kenyan mentor, Jumbam offers his advice with good humor and rapier wit.

It is good to have these two sages in my head as I try to draw conclusions from the myriad lessons I have been taught by the nurses, doctors, social workers, counselors, agribusiness experts, microfinance officials, PR partitioners, and the many patients and clients sitting somewhere waiting with me who were kind enough to chat for a moment.

I was reminded to listen to these real experts by Bob Einterz, who learned similar lessons from Haitians, and from Joe Mamlin, who learned from Afghans. I have learned from dozens of journalists and professors I worked with in South Asia before turning my attention to East Africa. And from my Kenyan mentors, such as professors Obi Okumu-Bigambo, Charles Ochieng' Ong'ondo, and Abraham Kiprop Mulwo in Eldoret, I again learned that the *real* experts are the people who live their experience each day. I am just a reporter, telling other people's stories and listening as carefully as I can.

The stories I collected during the spring of 2019 came from two types of people at AMPATH: leaders and workers. These are not mutually exclusive terms. Every leader I talked to worked as a doctor or pharmacist treating patients on the hospital wards. To a person, leaders at MTRH, Moi University, and the consortium talked about the devotion of people who worked *with* them, not for them. Similarly, the staff workers I talked with and observed spoke regularly of their efforts to lead. The projects they were working on were established by people higher in the organization, but they said they felt a responsibility to lead those whom the projects were intended to assist. Pamela Were, a highly accomplished nurse, thought of herself as leading the team that traveled to Sori for a screening clinic just as much as the doctor who headed the program. Kenneth Malaba worked on initiatives created by leaders of the Safety Net, but at the session he helped organize in Kitale with Mustapha Ghulam, he was confident in leading lectures and urging the participants to learn from the foreign expert. Papa Anyara did not design the GISHE system of economic empowerment, but he led dozens of the community savings groups and oversaw dozens of trainers who lead their own GISHE and other community groups. A hierarchy of authority that separated leaders from workers was even harder to see at the Rafiki Centre. Edith Apondi was at the top of the organizational chart, but meetings with her staff were a far more collaborative and consensual process among counselors, nurses, phlebotomists, clinicians, data analysts, and social workers than a top-down directive. And it wasn't just these four places where I saw this kind of duality, where workers were leaders and leaders were workers. It was also in the responses I received from nearly a quarter of those who get a paycheck from AMPATH. The stories told by the leaders in chapter 8 are remarkably similar to the stories told by workers in chapters 4, 5, 6, and 7.

Folks Work Together to Lead Their Community into the Future

All this must sound Pollyannish to anyone who has skipped from the introduction to the conclusion of this book. No organization the size and age of AMPATH is all clever harmony and sweet melody. There have been periods of discord and voices of dissension. AMPATH has made mistakes, and the leaders I interviewed admitted it, but very few workers let on that there were or had ever been any problems. Maybe folks I talked with were reticent to tell me about the downside because I was a guest in their country, perhaps even someone whose report could influence the donors that underwrite some of the projects they work with. I certainly gave everyone I talked to an opportunity to gripe and complain. What I heard was minor even though I could sometimes see room for complaint myself. A *mzungu* is more sensitive to power outages, broken toilets, rutted roads, noisy streets, and most certainly the more liberal definition of punctuality in Kenya. But no one complained about these trifles. The work was their focus. The mission was paramount.

I had anticipated this sense of mission because I had read so much of the research AMPATH generated about itself. Hundreds of articles in academic publications written by teams of Kenyans and North Americans have documented both the successes and limitations of the many projects taken up since the start of the IU-Kenya Partnership. They detail efforts at medical training, nutrition, and economic empowerment in addition to studies of disease treatment and prevention ranging from HIV/AIDS to cancer to hypertension to sickle cell. But the article I was most curious about before my sabbatical in 2019 was a 2007 study led by Tom Inui and conducted by a long list of Kenyan and Hoosier leaders who had for twenty years worked alongside the organization's staff workers. In a series of interviews, they determined that staffers worked as if they were responding to a calling of service.

When I was out reporting, I was listening for confirmation of the insights Tom and his colleagues discovered a decade earlier during a time when HIV was still a raging health emergency demanding urgent attention. Was the goodwill toward AMPATH and the devotion to the mission they identified something born of an emergency response, or was it something more endemic to the academic model?

My approach to answering that question was multimethodological. I observed carefully, documenting my observations with a camera and confirming the validity of my photographic depiction by asking those under my gaze whether I had it right. I interviewed both leaders and workers, wrote up their stories, and then asked each one to read what I had said and tell me where I had gone wrong. Again, maybe there was some deference to the old professor, but everyone said I had listened well and was portraying them as they really were. I think my previous experience teaching students from IU and Moi combined

with my study of the research reports the organization produced allowed me to see with a perspective that's more attuned to Kenya than someone without a history of working alongside professors and students at Moi and chatting with strangers on the streets for more than a decade. But to further confirm my observations, I also used a social science method to gauge the attitudes of a much larger sample than what I had observed in the oncology outreach team's work, the Safety Net operations, or the comprehensive care clinic for youth's programs. I asked everyone on the AMPATH payroll to take a survey to help me understand.

AMPATH workers who responded professed a commitment to the organization, found satisfaction in the work, believed the work they did was meaningful, and understood their motivation as driven by a desire to serve their community and nation. This was not by small margins. The key finding was that 93 percent of the staffers indicated they found a high level of meaning in their work, 89 percent were highly satisfied with their job, and 86 percent were highly committed to AMPATH as an organization. These statistics support contentions by MTRH CEO Aruasa and AMPATH chief of party Kimaiyo that the academic model has resulted in dramatically higher rates of staff retention than is typical in Kenya and the developing world. This is borne out when the overall average of 46 percent job satisfaction in studies conducted elsewhere in Kenya is compared with AMPATH's 89 percent level of job satisfaction. The very high levels of satisfaction my survey showed are not common across the country, and the academic model is likely the reason. Please see chapter 10's discussion of the survey results and the comments by staffers speaking to motivation, including a senior technical officer who encapsulated the survey's statistical results most poetically: "I believe my work and my purpose are intricately linked. Like a signature is to a painter, so is work to me. It is a reflection of who I am and why I am on this earth."

What I saw and heard led me to conclude that the people of AMPATH understand themselves as a part of something good. They see themselves on a mission to cure the sick, help the needy, and build a community that can take care of itself. They do this by building relationships among themselves and with their communities. They have taken the AMPATH motto to heart, and they are Leading with Care. I have come to understand that this means they care for others. The first thing is to care—not to treat, test, survey, or administer. Those are important, but first they care. They care enough to come back again and again, to go door to door, to meet with people in their churches and farm fields and neighborhoods. They care enough to listen, to remember, to sympathize, and to help their patients and clients find a solution. They sit with members of GISHE groups, Chama cha MamaToto groups, dairy cooperatives, county extension officers, rural clinic workers, street children, village elders, school groups, and anyone else who may provide them with insight into the aspirations of the community. Leading with Care starts with listening and ends with collaboration. As Laura Ruhl said, "It's often messy, and there's lots of drama sometimes, but it's much easier to get things done when people are talking and working together."

AMPATH people work together, and I don't think it unreasonable to say that they do so because they are answering a call to service. Tom heard the workers say this in 2007. I heard it again and again. Kenyans are a deeply religious people. They believe in harambee, the power of cooperation, and that a major part of being a good and moral person is acting in concert for the common good.

They are called to do this by a higher power. The work is their obligation to each other as Kenyans. This is obvious to every Kenyan. It is right there on the country's national coat of arms. It is the open secret to their national liberation and their national success.

Harambee

The word *harambee* is the national motto and it means "Let us all pull together." Mwende Mutuli Musau very nicely said that "it encompasses a concept of placing the group before the individual. For us Kenyans, a harambee represents an unwritten law of generosity, and regardless of class, ethnic group, gender, or religious background, we will lend a hand to assist anyone in need" (2020). There is also a thing called a harambee and it is representative of this larger concept that Musau speaks of. Broadly speaking, a harambee can be anything from a fundraising event to emotional support to a simple favor. "Whenever an individual is facing a significant rite of passage or life event—such as a wedding, educational opportunity, serious illness or a relative's funeral—and needs help, they will contact an elder family member or tribal leader. This leader will then call a meeting with other elders, and if the issue is deemed significant enough to warrant the strength of the community, they will share the issue with the individual's family, friends and co-workers and organize a harambee. Those in attendance often contribute money, services or emotional and physical support" according to Musau (2020).

Harambee is given without expectation of return. It is for the individual in need, but it is for the community as well. Harambee pulled the various tribal groups of Kenya together and pushed the British out in 1963. It pulled them together again to build a modern society after the colonials were gone. It constructed hospitals and universities, bridges and roads, houses and farms. Harambee today is part of every community event, from births to weddings to funerals. For *wazungu*, it is also infectious. Long-term residents from North America get swept up in it. I have donated money, time, and attention to harambee, and afterward I always feel like I am included in something lovely. I feel like I am part of a relationship that is without definition. I am always surprised by who contributes, how much and how little, and how great the expressions of gratitude are by those who receive—and also by those who give.

But I am no longer surprised by the way AMPATH works. I have never read anything about the partnership that has mentioned harambee, but I see evidence of it everywhere. I suspect Haroun Mengech saw it when Hoosiers came to visit Moi University in 1998 and that Joe, Sarah Ellen, Bob, Charlie, and Dave saw it too. The Hoosiers were ready to give without expectation of return. They were ready to join the harambee. Building a medical school was worthy. Everyone contributed what they could—Kenyans and Hoosiers according to their ability. They pulled together then, and they have pulled together along with others from the US and Canada for three decades now, through economic stress, tribal discord, and viral pandemic. Harambee built relationships that have endured long enough that the leaders can retire and their protégés can pull the weight they once lifted. Harambee will deliver the country to population health.

And harambee has started to spread the academic model beyond the Great Rift Valley. As I conclude this book, a few former Hoosiers who learned how to pull together while in Eldoret are now Leading with Care in West Africa and northern Mexico. Harambee is also spreading to other parts of Kenya. For years I myself asked why there were not AMPATHs elsewhere. Now it looks like there will be.

Dr. Rajesh "Raj" Vedanthan was the AMPATH Consortium's medicine team leader in 2005. I got to sit with him at the Siam Restaurant the first week I was in Eldoret during sabbatical. I asked him why AMPATH had not been replicated, and he said, "We are working on that now." It was why he was in town. By "we" he meant a team he headed at the Section for Global Health in New York University's Grossman School of Medicine. Later in the spring, Raj traveled to northern Ghana with Joe and Bob. They found willing partners at the University for Development Studies in Tamale and at the Tamale Teaching Hospital, particularly Dr. Francis Abantanga, then dean of the university's medical school. According to Raj, AMPATH Ghana aims to improve the health of the population in and around Tamale, develop insights that can be applied in other geographic areas of the country, inform national health policy, and generate lessons that that are relevant for other low-resource settings worldwide.

Tim Mercer was the AMPATH Consortium's medicine team leader from 2015 to 2017. I didn't get to know him then because IU had embargoed student travel to Eldoret during those years and I was in Uganda instead. I did get to meet him and his team while on sabbatical, however. Like Raj, he came to Eldoret in March 2019 to meet with Kimaiyo, Aruasa, Joe, Bob, and other leaders to discuss a replication of AMPATH. Tim had recently been named director of global health at the Dell Medical School at the University of Texas. He and his dean, Dr. Clay Johnston, wanted to establish a long-term, mutually beneficial, bilateral partnership with a medical school in Mexico to engage across the trifold academic mission of service, teaching, and research to strengthen health systems and improve health outcomes for low-income people. They had found partners at Benemerita Universidad Autonoma de Puebla School of Medicine in central Mexico and were building the relationships that have always sustained AMPATH in Kenya.

These two replications were described to me with great pride by Bob Einterz just as he was stepping down from his leadership of the consortium. They represent the hope that people pulling together in friendship following an academic model based on Leading with Care can help people throughout the developing world achieve self-sustaining healthcare systems that secure the health of the community and build the capacity of the country. One of the final acts of harambee that Bob committed on his way out was to secure multimillion-dollar grants to support each of these projects, with no expectation of return for himself or even his partners in Kenya.

The simple conclusion is that AMPATH's model works very well in the Eldoret region, and the best speculation is that it will work elsewhere too. It may even work well in other parts of Kenya. The Kenya Ministry of Health increasingly thinks of AMPATH as a model for the development of healthcare systems in other parts of the country. Several Kenyan leaders at AMPATH told me the partnership was seen as more innovative and more responsive to changing conditions than the rest of the country's systems and that national leaders wanted folks in Eldoret to join with other regions somewhat like the North Americans were spreading the academic model to Ghana and Mexico.

In August 2019, AMPATH was contracted by USAID to take over HIV care and related activities in Turkana County. It is the country's largest county by area, extending down the Great Rift Valley to Uganda, South Sudan, and Ethiopia. "We want AMPATH Plus to emphasize capacity building, to provide technical assistance, and support our county and sub-county teams to do their work. All activities should be carried out jointly so that our teams can learn and be ready when AMPATH Plus leaves Turkana," stated Dr. GilChrist Lokoel, the county's director of health (Keter 2019, 1). AMPATH's Sylvester Kimaiyo was a teacher in Turkana before earning his medical degree and locating in Eldoret, and folks there were thrilled that their teacher would return. In Kenya, relationships with people run deep.

Everywhere I looked while in Eldoret, I saw people helping themselves. My interviews with leaders substantiated my assessment that the projects I had observed over the months I was making photographs were working, and the survey results I collected at the end of my time in Kenya confirmed that essentially all the staff executing these projects believed in them and saw benefits for their society. I also caught a glimpse into the future of AMPATH at the Rafiki Centre. Youths there were empowered by their embrace of their own culture, excited by their universal education, and enthusiastic about a future where they will defeat corruption and grow prosperity. The youths who graduate from Rafiki will become leaders in their community and forceful advocates for universal healthcare funded by the NHIF.

The Last Supper at IU House

Joe and Sarah Ellen Mamlin had dinner at the IU House as long-term residents for the final time on April 7, 2019. The cooks made a chicken dish, and at the end of the meal, as he always had, Joe went from table to table collecting bones he would feed to the three dogs that guarded the compound. My wife, Carol Kelly, asked Joe from across the room, "Do you have someone picked out who will collect the bones after you are gone?" He replied, "I do what I do as long as I can, and then others will do what they can do."

The people working for AMPATH now do what they do, and they do it very well. Some were influenced directly by Hoosiers like Joe and Bob, but all have been infected by the spirit of collaboration and commitment that they—Mengech, Kimaiyo, and so many others—infused into a partnership among a medical school, a hospital, and a consortium of *wazungu* who went to Africa looking for partners and found lifelong friends. The success of AMPATH is as simple as that. Friends doing what they can do to make the world a better place.

But that begs the question as to why they do this hard work. Bob Einterz said it best: "It is love."

Epilogue

I said I was lucky. Looking back from January 2022, as this book goes to press, I see the spring of 2019 as one of the best times to have been talking to AMPATH folks about their many successes. The population health initiative was in full bloom. The comprehensive nature of the project was being embraced by all parts of the partnership: MTRH, Moi University, the AMPATH Consortium, and the Kenyan Ministry of Health. It meshed perfectly with the national government's plans for expanding the National Hospital Insurance Fund, and pilot studies were showing that AMPATH's community health messaging strategies were persuading an impressively large percentage of people in the villages to sign up for improved healthcare via NHIF.

And then the COVID-19 pandemic appeared. AMPATH had originally been launched to fight a pandemic in the 2000s. Leading with Care soon came to mean caring for increasing numbers of people contracting HIV. In 2020, it would also mean testing and treating people contracting the coronavirus but especially working to prevent the spread of the virus using the public health communication methods learned during the earlier HIV/AIDS pandemic. Leaders at the MTRH, Moi, and the consortium began restructuring their operations to respond to the emergency immediately after Kenyan president Uhuru Kenyatta issued an executive order establishing a National Emergency Response Committee on Coronavirus on February 28, 2020. A few days later, on March 3, Adrian Gardner, the new director of IU Center for Global Health and the AMPATH Consortium, issued his first statement regarding the global threat from the coronavirus. He had settled into the corner office occupied by Bob Einterz less than a month earlier.

The Kenyan government had acted swiftly to impose quarantines and restrictions on movement into and throughout the country. The first confirmed case of COVID-19 in Kenya was diagnosed in Nairobi on March 13, 2020, and by the end of the month, all the North Americans had left Eldoret for homes in North America. In an email to the consortium members, Gardner said, "It is, sadly, perhaps the first time in our thirty-year partnership that no North American faculty member has been on the ground in Kenya for an extended period of time."

And then, on April 6, the first case was diagnosed in Eldoret (Ndanyi 2020). AMPATH had used the weeks prior to establish a multidisciplinary task force, create a 24-7 hotline, train healthcare workers, set up isolation units, assemble supplies, establish protocols for screening and testing, and prepare the medical infrastructure to treat patients. Before that first positive case was detected, the MTRH had screened more than 105,000 people.

Sylvester Kimaiyo worked with USAID to modify AMPATH operations in light of COVID-19 by reducing HIV clinic visits by about 90 percent and by modifying the Differentiated Care and Community Model so patients could pick up their ARVs even during the lockdown that kept people off the streets of western Kenya for much of the spring and summer. GISHE groups began meeting virtually using their mobile phones. The Rafiki Centre building was converted into a COVID-19 isolation ward, and the adolescents moved into the basement of the AMPATH Centre. Public education efforts about masking, washing and sanitizing hands, observing physical distance, and avoiding public gatherings were organized and carried out by AMPATH population health workers across the region.

By August 31 there had been 33,794 confirmed cases and 572 deaths from COVID-19 in Kenya and 94,196 confirmed cases and 3,263 deaths in Indiana, which has about one-seventh the population (Johns Hopkins Coronavirus Resource Center 2020). Kenya and AMPATH had responded effectively to the epidemic. President Kenyatta ended the national curfew by summer's end, and international flights into the country resumed. IU's team leaders, Drs. Caitrin Kelly and Dan Guiles, arrived in Eldoret in mid-October 2020 and were warmly welcomed by the friends who had missed them.

Earlier in the summer, Indiana University's president, Michael McRobbie, had formed a Medical Response Team for COVID-19 to prepare all eight campuses for the return of students in the fall. The medical school's Dr. Aaron Carroll was placed in charge of mitigation testing, and AMPATH's Adrian Gardner headed the contact-tracing effort.

In a January 2021 article in *The Atlantic*, Carroll wrote about how some American universities had figured out how to diagnose their populations and control outbreaks. IU had been one of them (Carroll 2021). Transmission on campus was far lower than at peer universities that had not instituted mass testing and tracing programs. He credited lessons learned from the public health messaging campaigns conducted by AMPATH in Eldoret for part of IU's success. The work of AMPATH doctors, nurses, social workers, economic-empowerment officers, and community health volunteers during the public health response to HIV and other contagious outbreaks in Kenya had helped Hoosiers keep their campus relatively safe compared to the surrounding communities in Indiana.

By the spring, more and more Hoosiers and other members of the AMPATH Consortium were traveling to and living in Eldoret, working in the MTRH alongside their Kenyan colleagues and generally resuming the important work that had been interrupted at the onset of the epidemic. A mass vaccination campaign began in March as the number of cases and deaths continued to climb, though it never raged in Kenya the way it had in the US.

The work of public safety had been conducted at the highest levels of governance in support of the healthcare community—with impressive consistency. When case levels rose, measures were taken by the various county governments to tamp them down by setting curfews, closing schools, or taking other restrictive measures. As cases nationwide began to rise in the summer, President Kenyatta on August 18 again issued national containment guidelines that included another nationwide curfew from eight at night to four in the morning and the closing of all schools and universities. The government at the same time announced substantial tax relief to low-income earners and millions in sizable allocations to vulnerable groups, including the elderly and orphans, to assist them during the emergency. And then on October 20, in a nationally televised address, Kenyatta lifted the curfew and said, "It is now time to shift our focus from survival to co-existing with the disease." It was on Mashujaa Day or "Heroes Day," the public holiday honoring Kenyans who contributed to the country's independence struggle (*Saturday Standard* 2021).

AMPATH had also shifted its focus back to population health efforts and replication of the model in Mexico and Ghana. In November AMPATH partners were awarded another round of PEPFAR/USAID funding grants. The AMPATH Plus name will be retired and the new awards will bear the names USAID AMPATH Uzima, USAID Dumisha Afya and USAID 4TheChild. All of the new awards will continue for five years and total more than USD $120 million. While the geographic footprint of AMPATH's HIV program has changed over time, much of western Kenya has benefited from AMPATH's efforts in HIV prevention and treatment, chronic diseases management, economic empowerment, and other supportive

projects. The work was interrupted by the latest epidemic to confront healthcare workers in Kenya, but it continues nevertheless.

As this book goes to production on January 1, 2022 (many times delayed by hardships brought on by the pandemic), 5,378 Kenyans have died of COVID-19 and 825,536 Americans have died of the exact same virus. The average death rate in Kenya is 10 per 100,000 population whereas the death rate in the United States is 251 per 100,000. The vaccination rate is 7.8 percent in Kenya and 63 percent in the US. The difference in mortality rates is startling. I don't know why it is so great. Researchers at AMPATH and the Regenstrief Institute and other public health experts amid the consortium membership may someday come up with explanations for the difference. As for me, I like to think that the lessons learned by Kenyans during their horrific AIDS epidemic are the reason they now trust public health officials. I think government officials, healthcare leaders, and the general populace learned something very valuable about how to provide clear messaging to a public that is responsive and able to come together to protect itself. I think AMPATH is a major part of the reason people in Kenya are keeping as safe as they have been. I don't know this for a fact, but it makes sense to me based on my long observation of people there.

What I do know is that through it all, the partnership has remained strong. Just as it had to adjust its orientation to healthcare twenty years ago when AIDS swept the globe, today it is adjusting again as the COVID-19 pandemic becomes the pressing priority. Lessons learned during more than thirty years of collaboration continue to sustain the health and well-being of people in Africa and North America, and someday soon even more of these friends will be together again, building a population health system robust enough to respond to the next emergency, as well as the daily needs of Kenyans.

REFERENCES

Agence France-Presse. 2019. "Eliud Kipchoge Busts Mythical Two-Hour Marathon Barrier." *Daily Nation*, October 12, 2019.

Allen, Luke, Julianne Williams, Nick Townsend, Bente Mikkelsen, Nia Roberts, Charlie Foster, and Kremlin Wickramasinghe. 2017. "Socioeconomic Status and Non-Communicable Disease Behavioural Risk Factors in Low-Income and Lower-Middle-Income Countries: A Systematic Review." *Lancet Global Health* 5, no. 3 (March): e277–89.

Allen, Natalie J., and John P. Meyer. 1990. "The Measurement and Antecedents of Affective, Continuance and Normative Commitment to the Organization." *Journal of Occupational Psychology* 63 (1): 1–18.

American Association for Public Opinion Research. n.d. "Standard Definitions: Final Dispositions of Case Codes and Outcome Rates for Surveys." Last revised 2016. Accessed December 30, 2021. https://www.aapor.org/Standards -Ethics/Standard-Definitions-(1).aspx.

Baruch, Yehuda, and Brooks C. Holtom. 2008. "Survey Response Rate Levels and Trends in Organizational Research." *Human Relations* 61 (8): 1139–60.

Bowling, Nathan A., and Gregory D. Hammond. 2008. "A Meta-Analytic Examination of the Construct Validity of the Michigan Organizational Assessment Questionnaire Job Satisfaction Subscale." *Journal of Vocational Behavior* 73, no. 1 (August): 63–77.

Brownie, Sharon, and Elizabeth Oywer. 2016. "Health Professionals in Kenya: Strategies to Expand Reach and Reduce Brain Drain of Psychiatric Nurses and Psychiatrists." *BJPsych International* 13 (3): 55–58.

Bush, George W. 2003. "State of the Union." White House Archives. January 28, 2003.

Cairns, Gus. 2013. "The Diminished Self—HIV and Self-Stigma." NAM. June 25, 2013.

Cammann, Cortlandt, Mark Fichman, Douglas Jenkins, and John Klesh. 1979. *The Michigan Organizational Assessment Questionnaire*. Ann Arbor: University of Michigan.

Carroll, Aaron. 2021. "The Colleges That Took the Pandemic Seriously." *The Atlantic*, January 31, 2021. https://www .theatlantic.com/ideas/archive/2021/01/colleges-took -pandemic-seriously/617879/.

Duffy, Ryan D., and Bryan J. Dik. 2013. "Research on Calling: What Have We Learned and Where Are We Going?" *Journal of Vocational Behavior* 83, no. 3 (December): 428–36.

Duffy, Ryan D., Jessica W. England, Richard P. Douglass, Kelsey L. Autin, and Blake A. Allan. 2017. "Perceiving a Calling and Well-Being: Motivation and Access to Opportunity as Moderators." *Journal of Vocational Behavior* 98 (February): 127–37.

Einterz, Robert. 2015. "A Case Study in Global Health Harnessing the Power of Partnerships." *American Outlook* (Fall): 5–16. https://www.sagamoreinstitute.org/wp-content /uploads/2020/03/IU-Kenya-Medical-Partnership.pdf.

Esarey, Logan. 1924. *History of Indiana from Its Exploration to 1922*. Edited by Kate Milner Rabb and William Herschell. Dayton, OH: Dayton Historical Pub. Co.

Gathura, Gatonye. 2019. "US Cuts Funding to Kenya's AIDS War, Cites Sharp Drop in Cases." *Standard*, August 18, 2019.

Geib, George W. 1981. *Indianapolis, Hoosiers' Circle City*. American Portrait Series. Tulsa, OK: Continental Heritage Press.

Graboyes, Melissa. 2014. "Introduction: Incorporating Medical Research into the History of Medicine in East Africa." *International Journal of African Historical Studies* 47 (3): 379–98.

———. 2015. *Experiment Must Continue: Medical Research and Ethics in East Africa, 1940–2014*. Perspectives on Global Health. Athens: Ohio University Press.

Heller, Jean. 1972. "Syphilis Victims in U.S. Study Went Untreated for 40 Years." *New York Times*, July 26, 1972, 1.

Herbert, Bob. 2001. "In America; Refusing to Save Africans." *New York Times*, June 11, 2001.

Ighobor, Kingsley. 2017. "Diagnosing Africa's Medical Brain Drain." *United Nations Africa Renewal*, March 2017. https:// www.un.org/africarenewal/magazine/december-2016 -march-2017/diagnosing-africa%E2%80%99s-medical -brain-drain.

Indiana University. 2007. "$60 Million USAID Grant Goes to Indiana and Moi Universities' AMPATH Program to Combat AIDS in Kenya." News release. November 19, 2007.

Inui, Thomas S., Winston[e] M. Nyandiko, Sylvester N. Kimaiyo, Richard M. Frankel, Tadeo Muriuki, Joseph J. Mamlin, Robert M. Einterz, and John E. Sidle. 2007. "AMPATH: Living Proof That No One Has to Die from HIV." *Journal of General Internal Medicine* 22, no. 12 (December): 1745–50.

Johns Hopkins Coronavirus Resource Center. 2020. "Mortality Analyses." Accessed August 31, 2020. https://coronavirus .jhu.edu/data/mortality.

———. 2022. "Mortality Analyses." Accessed January 1, 2022. https://coronavirus.jhu.edu/data/mortality.

Jones, James H. 1993. *Bad Blood: The Tuskegee Syphilis Experiment*. New and expanded ed. New York: Free Press.

Jumbam, Desmond T. 2020. "How (Not) to Write about Global Health." *BMJ Global Health* 5 (7): e003164.

Kasper, Jennifer, and Francis Bajunirwe. 2012. "Brain Drain in Sub-Saharan Africa: Contributing Factors, Potential Remedies and the Role of Academic Medical Centres." *Archives of Disease in Childhood* 97, no. 11 (November): 973–79.

Kasprowicz, Victoria, Denis Chopera, Kim Darley Waddilove, Mark A. Brockman, Jill Gilmour, Eric Hunter, William Kilembe, Etienne Karita, Simani Gaseitsiwe, Eduard J. Sanders, and Thumbi Ndung'u. 2020. "African-led Health Research and Capacity Building: Is It Working?" *BMC Public Health* 20 (1): 1104–14.

Keeter, Scott, Courtney Kennedy, Dimock Michael, Jonathan Best, and Craighill Peyton. 2006. "Gauging the Impact of Growing Nonresponse on Estimates from a National RDD Telephone Survey." *Public Opinion Quarterly* 70 (5): 759–79.

Kennedy, Courtney, and Hannah Hartig. 2019. "Response Rates in Telephone Surveys Have Resumed Their Decline." Pew Research Center. February 27, 2019. https://www .pewresearch.org/fact-tank/2019/02/27/response-rates-in -telephone-surveys-have-resumed-their-decline/.

Keter, Sammy. 2019. "AMPATH Plus Hits the Ground Running in Turkana County." AMPATH. November 22, 2019. https://www.ampathkenya.org/news-blog-feed/2019 /11/30/ampathplus-hits-the-ground-running-in-turkana -county.

Koech, Emily, Chloe A. Teasdale, Chunhui Wang, Ruby Fayorsey, Terezah Alwar, Irene N. Mukui, Mark Hawken, and Elaine J. Abrams. 2014. "Characteristics and Outcomes of HIV-Infected Youth and Young Adolescents Enrolled in HIV Care in Kenya." *AIDS* 28 (18): 2729–38.

Kokonya, Donald A., John M. Mburu, Dammas M. Kathuku, Ndetei DM, Adam H. Adam, Desire A. Nshimirimana, Phocas S. Biraboneye, and Louise M. Kpoto. 2014. "Burnout Syndrome among Medical Workers at Kenyatta National

Hospital (KNH), Nairobi, Kenya." *Journal of Psychiatry* (South Africa) 17, no. 6 (January): 14–20.

Loscocco, Karyn A., and Anne R. Roschelle. 1991. "Influences on the Quality of Work and Nonwork Life: Two Decades in Review." *Journal of Vocational Behavior* 39, no. 2 (January): 182–225.

Malaba, Kenneth, Robert Otuya, and Erenst Saina. 2018. "Social Factors Influencing Adoption of Grain Amaranth/Maize Intercrop among Small Holder Farmers in Kiminini, Kenya." *African Journal of Education, Science and Technology* 4, no. 4 (December): 48–57.

Mcintosh, Ian S., and Eunice Kamaara. 2016. "AMPATH: A Strategic Partnership in Kenya." In *Global Perspectives on Strategic International Partnerships: A Guide to Building Sustainable Academic Linkages*, edited by Clare Banks, Birgit Siebe-Herbig, and Karin Norton. New York: Institute of International Education, 255–65.

Mercer, Tim, Adrian Gardner, Benjamin Andama, Cleophas Chesoli, Astrid Christoffersen-Deb, Jonathan Dick, Robert Einterz et al. 2018. "Leveraging the Power of Partnerships: Spreading the Vision for a Population Health Care Delivery Model in Western Kenya." *Globalization and Health* 14, no. 1 (May): 44–55.

Meslin, Eric M., David Ayuku, and Edwin Were. 2014. "'Because It Was Hard . . .': Some Lessons Developing a Joint IRB between Moi University (Kenya) and Indiana University (USA)." *American Journal of Bioethics* 14 (5): 17–19.

Ministry of Health. 2015a. *Devolved HRM Policy Guidelines on Human Resources for Health*. Nairobi, Kenya.

———. 2015b. *Kenya Health Workforce Report: The Status of Healthcare Professionals in Kenya, 2015*. Nairobi, Kenya.

Muraguri, Mwangi. 2015. "Stop Brain Drain in Health Sector, Kenya Urged." *Standard*, September 7, 2015.

Musau, Mwende Mutuli. 2020. "Harambee: The Rule of Generosity That Rules Kenya." BBC. October 5, 2020. http://www.bbc.com/travel/story/20201004-harambee-the-kenyan-word-that-birthed-a-nation?ocid=global_travel_rss.

National AIDS Control Council (NACC). 2018. *Kenya HIV Estimates Report 2018*. Nairobi, Kenya: NACC.

Ndanyi, Mathews. 2020. "Eldoret's First Patient Had No Symptoms during Her Quarantine." *Star*, April 8, 2020.

Ndege, George O. 2001. *Health, State, and Society in Kenya*. Rochester, NY: University of Rochester Press.

Ogaji, Ikoni J., Titus M. Kahiga, Onesmus W. Gachuno, and Julius W. Mwangi. 2016. "Development of Pharmacy Education in Kenya Universities to Date." *African Journal of Pharmacy and Pharmacology* 10 (18): 385–92.

Ojakaa, David, Susan Olango, and Jordan Jarvis. 2014. "Factors Affecting Motivation and Retention of Primary Health Care Workers in Three Disparate Regions in Kenya." *Human Resources for Health* 12, no. 1 (June): 33.

Oketch, Angela. 2019. "Burnout a Ticking Time Bomb among Medical Staff." *Daily Nation*, April 6, 2019.

Otieno, Dorothy. 2016. "Overwork Leading to Burn-Out among Kenya's Nurses." *Daily Nation*, May 15, 2016.

Pantelic, Marija, Mark Boyes, Lucie Cluver, and Franziska Meinck. 2017. "HIV, Violence, Blame and Shame: Pathways of Risk to Internalized HIV Stigma among South African Adolescents Living with HIV." *Journal of the International AIDS Society* 20 (1): 21771.

Parsons, Timothy H. 2012. *The Rule of Empires: Those Who Built Them, Those Who Endured Them, and Why They Always Fall*. New York: Oxford University Press.

Phillips, Clifton J. 1968. *Indiana in Transition: The Emergence of an Industrial Commonwealth, 1880–1920*. Indianapolis: Indiana Historical Bureau and Indiana Historical Society.

Poppe, Annelien, Elena Jirovsky, Claire Blacklock, Pallavi Laxmikanth, Shabir Moosa, Jan De Maeseneer, Ruth Kutalek, and Wim Peersman. 2014. "Why Sub-Saharan African Health Workers Migrate to European Countries That Do Not Actively Recruit: A Qualitative Study Post-Migration." *Global Health Action* 7: 24071–71.

Quigley, Fran. 2009. *Walking Together, Walking Far: How a U.S. and African Medical School Partnership Is Winning the Fight against HIV/AIDS*. Bloomington: Indiana University Press.

Republic of Kenya. 1994. *Development Plan, 1994–1996*. Nairobi, Kenya: Government Printer.

Rosso, Brent D., Kathryn H. Dekas, and Amy Wrzesniewski. 2010. "On the Meaning of Work: A Theoretical Integration and Review." *Research in Organizational Behavior* 30:91–127.

Saturday Standard. 2021. "President Uhuru Kenyatta's Mashujaa Day Full Speech." October 20, 2021.

Serwadda, David, Roy D. Mugerwa, Nelson K. Sewankambo, Anthony Lwegaba, John Wilson Carswell, George B. Kirya, Anne C. Bayley et al. 1985. "Slim Disease: A New Disease in Uganda and Its Association with HTLV-III Infection." *Lancet* 2, no. 8460 (October): 849–52.

Steger, Michael F., Bryan J. Dik, and Ryan D. Duffy. 2012. "Measuring Meaningful Work: The Work and Meaning Inventory (WAMI)." *Journal of Career Assessment* 20 (3): 322–37.

Tsofa, Benjamin, Catherine Goodman, Lucy Gilson, and Sassy Molyneux. 2017. "Devolution and Its Effects on Health Workforce and Commodities Management—Early Implementation Experiences in Kilifi County, Kenya." *International Journal for Equity in Health* 16 (1): 169–82.

Turissini, Matthew, Tim Mercer, Jenny Baenziger, Lukoye Atwoli, Robert Einterz, Adrian Gardner, Debra Litzelman, and Paul Ayuo. 2020. "Developing Ethical and Sustainable Global Health Educational Exchanges for Clinical Trainees: Implementation and Lessons Learned from the 30-Year Academic Model Providing Access to Healthcare (AMPATH) Partnership." *Annals of Global Health* 86 (1): 137–46.

Uyoga, Sophie, Alex W. Macharia, George Mochamah, Carolyne M. Ndila, Gideon Nyutu, Johnstone Makale, Metrine Tendwa et al. 2019. "The Epidemiology of Sickle Cell Disease in Children Recruited in Infancy in Kilifi, Kenya: A Prospective Cohort Study." *Lancet Global Health* 7 (10): e1458–66.

Wainaina, Binyavanga. 2005. "How to Write About Africa." *Granta* 92 (Winter). https://granta.com/how-to-write-about-africa/.

Washington, Harriet A. 2006. *Medical Apartheid: The Dark History of Medical Experimentation on Black Americans from Colonial Times to the Present.* 1st ed. New York: Doubleday.

Were, Pamela, Constance Tenge, Naftali Busakhala, and Patrick Loehrer. 2006. "Developing Oncology Outreach Services in Western Kenya Region." Paper presented at the World Cancer Congress, Washington, DC.

Willinger, Ulrike, Andreas Hergovich, Michaela Schmoeger, Matthias Deckert, Susanne Stoettner, Iris Bunda, Andrea Witting et al. 2017. "Cognitive and Emotional Demands of Black Humour Processing: The Role of Intelligence, Aggressiveness and Mood." *Cognitive Processing* 18, no. 2 (May): 159–67.

Willis-Shattuck, Mischa, Posy Bidwell, Steve Thomas, Laura Wyness, Duane Blaauw, and Prudence Ditlopo. 2008. "Motivation and Retention of Health Workers in Developing Countries: A Systematic Review." *BMC Health Services Research* 8 (December): 247–55.

Wrzesniewski, Amy, Clark McCauley, Paul Rozin, and Barry Schwartz. 1997. "Jobs, Careers, and Callings: People's Relations to Their Work." *Journal of Research in Personality* 31, no. 1 (March): 21–33.

Yamin, Alicia Ely, and Allan Maleche. 2017. "Realizing Universal Health Coverage in East Africa: The Relevance of Human Rights." *BMC International Health and Human Rights* 17:21.

INDEX

Page numbers in *italics* refer to illustrations

17, 19, 151; medical, 17, 20, 30, 130, 134, 142, 143; public, 137, 192; sex education, 104. *See also* farmers: education of; Ministry of Education (MoE)

Einterz, Bob, 17, 20, 24, 27, 44, 67, 69, 112, 113, 116, 118, 124, 132, 135, 142, 144, 147, 155, 158, 160–65, 184, 188, 189, 191

Einterz, Ellen, 67

Einterz, Lea Anne, 144, 162

Eldoret, 6, 7, 8, 9, 10, 14, 16, 17, 18, 19–20, 21, 22, 23, 27, 28, 29, 32, 37, 43, 44, 49, 52, 56, 59, 61, 62, 67, 70, 72, 73, 75, 76, 77, 78, 80, 83, 84, 85, 88, 93, 98, 102, 112, 114, 115, 116, 118, 119, 120, 121, 122, 125, 126, 128, 130, 132, 134, 135, 137, 138, 139, 141, 142, 144, 146, 148, 150, 151, 152, 154, 155, 156, 157, 158, 160, 161, 162, 163, 170, 174, 175, 176, 179, 180, 181, 184, 187, 188, 192

Eldoret District Hospital, 20, 122

Eldoret University, 47

Elgon View Hospital, 20

emigration, 30, 31, 148

empowerment, 11, 99, 112, 113, 115, 138, 143, 171, 180, 188; economic, 14, 49, 51, 61, 160, 170, 171, 184, 185, 192, 193. *See also* group empowerment service providers (GESPs); Group Integrated Savings for Health and Empowerment (GISHE

Esamai, Fabian, 132, 142

Eskenazi Hospital, 163

ethics, 78, 173–74

Ethiopia, 8, 12, 188

Europe, 13, 16, 18, 21, 24, 31; Europeans, 6, 15–16, 19, 158

Everett, Julie, 148

family planning, 30, 162

Family Preservation Initiative (FPI), 40, 44, 48, 49, 51, 61, 62, 96, 102

farmers, 11, 61, 62, 64, 65–66, 72, 73; education of, 13, 29, 59, 61, 62, 72, 170; smallholder, 49, 61, 62, 63; subsistence, 128

farming, 18, 65; dairy, 63; farming practices, 29, 60, 62, 66; farming productivity, 62, 170

farms, 9, 11, 19, 28, 29, 42, 43, 49, 186, 187; small, 43, 65

food, 6, 23, 29, 51, 54, 56, 66, 96, 103; food security, 30, 49, 61, 128, 132. *See also* Corteva Agriscience (Dow Agriculture): Corteva Grows Food Security

Fore, Henrietta, 24

foundations, 23, 24, 30, 67, 68, 69, 113, 133, 156, 163. *See also individual foundation names*

funding, 16, 24, 28, 31, 52, 70, 113, 118, 119, 125, 128, 133, 139, 143, 146, 156, 160, 163, 170; funding agencies, 51, 119; government, 16, 24, 59, 129, 146

Fwamba, Margaret, 76

Gardner, Adrian, 7, 69, 120, 132, 133, 142, 147, 152, 154–58, 161, 191, 192

Gardner, Jessica, 152, 155

Gates Foundation, 30, 68

Ghana, 116, 160, 187, 188, 193

Ghulam, Mustafa, 59, 62, 63, 184

global health, 22, 28, 67, 70, 116, 135, 137, 152, 155, 158, 160, 162, 187. *See also* Indiana University Center for Global Health

government jobs, 59, 61

Graboyes, Melissa, 15, 16, 174

Gramelspacher, Gregory, 155

Gray, Nick, 69

Great Rift Valley, 5, 10, 15, 18, 49, 66, 79, 112, 141, 187, 188

group empowerment service providers (GESPs), 43, 44, 48, 52, 55

Group Integrated Savings for Health and Empowerment (GISHE), 37, 40, 41, 42–43, 44, 47, 48, 49, 51, 52, 53, 54, 55, 56, 61, 72, 143, 184, 186, 192

Guiles, Dan, 192

gynecology, 78, 121, 130

HAART and Harvest Initiative (HHI), 51

Haiti, 17–18, 162, 184

Hamm, Brad, 8

Hammond, Gregory D., 176

harambee (community self-help), 16, 186–87, 188

Hartig, Hannah, 177

Harvard School of Public Health, 155

Harvard University, 126, 155, 161

health workers, 6, 9, 29, 30, 31, 129, 133, 169, 170, 179, 180, 192, 193; community health workers (CHWs), 44, 82, 114, 143. *See also* doctors; nurses; retention: of staff

Heller, Jean, 173

hematology, 75

HIV, 8, 21, 72, 95, 102, 104, 106, 119, 122, 129, 137, 143, 150, 152, 155, 163, 185, 191, 192, 193; clinics, 23, 96, 119, 125, 192; deaths, 48; drugs, 23, 24, 69, 95, 151, 154; epidemic, 44, 113, 118, 129, 171; negative status, 94, 103, 122, 171; positive patients, 42, 44, 47, 49, 51–52, 54, 61, 67, 75, 83, 85, 87, 89, 90, 91, 93, 98, 116, 119, 122, 124, 125, 135, 137, 147, 151, 155, 170, 171; prevention, 24, 25, 68, 115, 119, 152, 193; rates, 24, 154; stigma, 23, 28, 90–91, 94, 99, 103, 137, 171; testing, 44, 93, 180; transmission of, 115, 122, 137; treatment, 44, 52, 67, 69, 70, 93, 96, 98, 102, 103, 113, 114, 115, 118, 122, 124, 125, 146, 150, 152, 171, 188, 193. *See also* AIDS; HIV/AIDS; prevention of mother-to-child transmission of HIV (PMTCT)

HIV/AIDS, 6, 7, 10, 13, 24, 25, 27, 132, 185; epidemic, 29, 112, 118, 122, 160, 161, 191; features of, 21; history of, 20–21; programs, 118; treatment, 23. *See also* AIDS; HIV

Hock Family Foundation, 28

holistic approach, 10, 17, 28, 29, 30, 51

Homa Bay, 77, 80

home testing and counseling (HTC), 51, 87

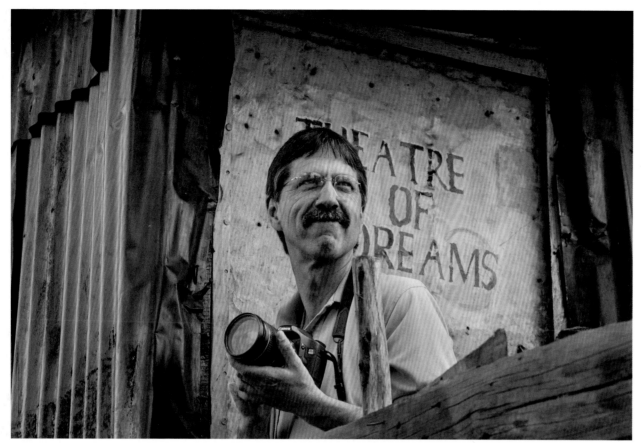

Photo by Noor Khamis, 2009

JAMES D. KELLY is Associate Professor and Director of Journalism
in the Media School at Indiana University Bloomington, where his work
focuses on photojournalism and healthcare reporting.